I0449587

The ProportionFit Diet
Orthopedic Edition

Count Cups, Not Calories

NICHOLAS J. MEYER, MD

Copyright © 2016 Nicholas J. Meyer, MD.

All rights reserved. No part of this book may be reproduced, stored, or transmitted by any means—whether auditory, graphic, mechanical, or electronic—without written permission of both publisher and author, except in the case of brief excerpts used in critical articles and reviews. Unauthorized reproduction of any part of this work is illegal and is punishable by law.

ISBN: 978-1-365-06922-2

The content of this book is the original work of Nicholas J. Meyer and has been adapted from *The ProportionFit Diet* to compliment a healthy diet and exercise. Twin Cities Orthopedics (TCO) does not explicitly or implicitly endorse the contents herein.

This book is intended as a reference for those interested in understanding the human diet; it is not a medical text or a replacement for a personal, professional medical opinion and should not be treated as such. It is designed to assist the reader in making informed decisions about his or her health but is not a substitute for a treatment that has been, or will be, prescribed by a doctor. Please consult with a doctor before instituting any drastic changes to your diet or if you suspect that you may have any medical conditions warranting evaluation.

Any mention of specific companies, products, organizations, departments, committees, administrations, or authorities does not imply endorsement by the author or publisher, nor does it imply that they endorse this book or the proportionfit.com website. All data contained herein is accurate to the knowledge of the author at the time of publication and any errors found herein are incidental and unintentional.

Because of the dynamic nature of the Internet, any web addresses or links contained in this book may have changed since publication and may no longer be valid. The views expressed in this work are solely those of the author and do not necessarily reflect the views of the publisher, and the publisher hereby disclaims any responsibility for them.

CONTENTS

Part II:
The ProportionFit Plan

PREFACE

This book is dedicated to everyone who struggles to be fit and to find a healthy weight. The goal of this book is to minimize that struggle by empowering the reader through knowledge and understanding. To borrow from a famous phrase, we will prove that the pen is mightier than the fork.

I would like to acknowledge and thank my loving and caring wife, Karen, and daughters, Ellie, Sonia, and Nina. Without their support and understanding, I could not have brought this to completion.

Additional thanks to Ben Kremer, Mark Russell, Precise Medical Technologies, Dr. Bob Meisterling, Paul Lewis Design, and registered dietician Jen Sletten for their thoughtful and honest input.

Thanks to Twin Cities Orthopedics for their vision, collaboration and assistance. As an organization, they understand the importance of health in the treatment of the whole patient. Special thanks to Kaitlyn Wahldick for the excellent cover design.

Finally, this book is written in the spirit of freedom, independence, understanding, self-determination, and seeking one's full potential. For, without these things, we would be imprisoned, dependent, ignorant, enslaved, and wasted in mind, body, and spirit.

Most people do not really want freedom, because freedom involves responsibility, and most people are frightened of responsibility.
—Sigmund Freud, *Civilization and Its Discontents*

INTRODUCTION

Freedom. While you may assume this book is about a diet, it is about more than that. It is about freedom: freedom to be obese, overweight, underweight, or anywhere in between. This book will provide an understanding as to why you are the weight you are and how, if you want, you can affect your weight. When you change the paradigm by which you view food and calories, you will see food differently and with elegant simplicity. What you do with that knowledge becomes an exercise in free will. I hope you will take this knowledge and combine it with the freedom you have been granted to make a positive impact in your life.

With bookshelves littered with multiple diet books, one might wonder: Why should I choose this book? The answer is simple: while others try to give you a simple, pain-free way to diet (which sadly does not exist), this book provides you with a simple, *realistic* way to diet and become healthier and happier. In other words, there may be some hunger involved (gasp!).

This is not about a special pill, extravagant meal plans, or somehow losing weight without a little sacrifice. This is about losing weight and maintaining an appropriate weight, becoming healthier, and achieving this goal without turning your lifestyle, your budget, or your sanity upside down. This diet system involves this book and a portion management tool (such as a measuring cup) of your choice. The book gives you some background knowledge and enlightenment to help you in your quest to achieve a healthy weight. The portion management tool will give you a visual and practical reminder to ensure an appropriate portion intake. It truly is that simple.

Why "ProportionFit"? The success of weight loss or healthy weight maintenance requires a combination of calorie intake *proportionate* to *the weight you want to be* along with physical fitness or exercise. This appropriate calorie intake is delivered by a number of *portions* appropriate for that goal weight. In this diet program, a portion is a cup of food, and the number of cups allowed daily is based simply on your body weight (either your goal weight or your current weight). By following these simple rules, you will find yourself more *fit*. In other words, eat proportionate portions to get fit or just get *ProportionFit!*

The use of a measuring cup as a simple and handy portion measurement tool is revolutionary in its simplicity. Combined with the knowledge of cup-sized portions and the appropriate volumes of food necessary for weight loss, The ProportionFit Diet will provide you with a simple, effective, and inexpensive system for losing weight and maintaining a healthy weight. It IS that simple.

PART I:

The Background

Where there is a will, there is a way.
—Author unknown, *New Monthly Magazine*, 1822

CHAPTER 1

Bottom Line Up Front

If you do not make it through this entire book, remember these key points because they are reinforced throughout the book and make the foundation for the ProportionFit concept:

1. On average, food contains approximately 280 calories per cup (8 ounces). The cup will be our universal portion.

2. The average person requires approximately 14 calories per pound daily to meet his or her daily calorie requirements (to maintain his or her current weight).

3. A deficit or surplus of 3,500 calories will either remove (if there's a deficit) or add (if there's a surplus) a pound to a person's weight over time.

4. A cup of food (remember: 280 calories) will provide the daily energy for about 20 pounds of body mass.

5. Thus a 200-pound person requires approximately 2,800 calories per day (at 14 calories per pound) and approximately

10 cups of food daily (equivalent to 2,800 calories) or one cup for every 20 pounds.

6. A balanced dietary intake of protein, fat, and carbohydrates is critical to a healthy and well-balanced diet.

7. As one's weight decreases, one's calorie requirements similarly decrease (remember: 14 calories per pound), leading to less weight loss over time despite the same limited consumption.

8. Hunger is the body's signal of a calorie deficit. It is not to be feared or avoided if attempting to lose weight. In fact, it is necessary and a sign of ongoing weight loss, if managed appropriately.

9. For every one cup daily deficit (in relation to current weight) the body will lose approximately a half pound weekly.

10. Once the goal weight is achieved, it is critical to consume only the number of cups necessary for that weight to maintain that weight.

11. Calories count, but counting cups is easier!

If you are what you eat, then your weight will be proportionate to your food intake (more on this later). Imagine: If you had eaten 10% less than you did over the entire last year, you would weigh approximately 10% less than you do right now. Since we cannot turn the clock back, changing your weight a year from now starts right *now*.

I, too, have struggled with weight loss. But I, and countless others, have succeeded using this system. My inspiration and ongoing commitment to helping others with weight loss stems from the pride and hope others have shared with me as they experience weight loss and improved health through these simple changes. Now it is your turn to be a success story by applying these ProportionFit principles.

Chapter One Bottom Line:

Your weight is defined by the volume of food consumed. That volume, if managed appropriately, can be used to lose weight and maintain a healthy weight. With The ProportionFit Diet, you will change only one thing with your diet: You will measure and quantify the volume of food consumed on a daily basis. That's the only change necessary. Until now, you likely have not paid attention to the exact volume of food you consume on a daily basis. Why? Because we have not been taught to do this. That changes today—based on science, actual results, and practicality. Read on for more.

The difference between a successful person and others is not a lack of strength, not a lack of knowledge, but rather a lack of will.
–Vince Lombardi

Testimonial:

"I joined the ProportionFit Diet program in July of 2014 after struggling with weight my whole life. I have tried numerous diet plans in the past and would lose weight and quickly gain it back again. I finally made the decision that it was time to try something structured and easy to follow. The ProportionFit Diet book is just that and has literally changed my life. I'm excited to say with measuring my portions and having a structured workout program through CrossFit, I have lost 80 pounds as of November 2015. I have more energy, I'm no longer in plus size clothing and I feel confident to tackle another 40 pounds to reach my ultimate goal of 100 pounds lost. Thank you Dr. Nick Meyer and the ProportionFit Diet!"

-Abby

CHAPTER 2

Shed the Victim Mentality before You Shed the Pounds

You are not a victim. The weight problem you and I have (or are trying to avoid) is not due to fast food. It is not due to your boss at work. It is not due to [insert whatever other excuse you may want to use]. It is due to too many calories going in and not enough calories being burned off by your system.

Why you put too many calories into your system is often multifactorial (see excuses above). However, the *act* of putting those calories in (i.e., feeding oneself) is a purposeful, deliberate act. No one is forcing you or me to place a doughnut in our mouths or to eat one more piece of pizza. Weight loss is not only gratifying for the purpose of losing weight but also empowering as you take control of your weight, your food intake, and your health.

We are constantly being told that we are victims of the supersized fast food meals, sugary sodas and juices, and too many carbs, fats, proteins, or whatever the current fad. While these factors add to the challenge of weight loss, they are not the reason for obesity.

To lose the weight, we need to discard the victim mentality and take charge of our health. This book and simple system should allow you to lose weight, control your weight, and maintain a healthy physique. Will you be hungry at times during this diet? Absolutely. Will it be a little painful at times to pass on the chocolate cake and free cookies at the school fair? Definitely. These acts, however simple, are pieces of the larger weight loss puzzle and lead to you taking charge of your health and leaving the other self-proclaimed victims of obesity to wallow in despair while you do something about it.

If you are overweight, obese, morbidly obese, or just interested in maintaining a healthy weight, the answer is simple: controlled caloric intake and exercise. This is the same message that has been touted for ages; the ProportionFit system makes it easier to follow and reinforces some simple principles.

Much of the inspiration for this system came from the comments made by gastric bypass patients I met in clinic. These patients lamented the fact that, had they been able to adhere to the limited intake they are now forced to follow post-operatively, they would have been able to lose the weight without the surgery. One of the goals of this system is to allow patients and other individuals another perspective on food intake and management.

Remember that we said this book was about freedom? Gastric bypass patients often lose the freedom to eat what they want. This is our attempt to bypass the bypass by empowering you with knowledge and inciting you to act for change. We've been told to cut calories and limit our intake, but this has been a tall order because of the complexity of calorie counting. We are left wondering: Cut how many calories? Limit our intake to what amount? What can I eat or what should I eat?

Eat this, not that? But how much of this should I eat? This system is so simple that anyone could follow it and succeed. No more excuses. No more victims. Only victors.

Chapter Two Bottom Line:

Most of us have not been properly educated in nutrition and caloric intake, and most government programs do not take a practical approach to weight-loss and a proper diet. By following the tenets of this book, you will be able to make one simple change to your dietary routine and effect your weight for the better. But, you are in charge. The success or failure of this system is defined by the adherence to the principles of the ProportionFit Diet. A wonderful illustration of this fact can be found in the results of those following the diet (see the "Track" tab at ProportionFit.com). For example, at the time of this publication, the average weight loss for those following the diet "exactly" or "fairly closely" at two months was 17.125 pounds, whereas those following the diet "somewhat" or "slightly" lost an average of 5.5 pounds.

You are what you eat.
— Nutritionist Victor Lindlahr

CHAPTER 3

The Ins and Outs of Caloric Balance

If you have ever asked yourself how you managed to gain weight over the years, the answer is exceedingly simple: more calories went in than were utilized by your body.

Imagine a train with a coal-burning steam engine. You have to shovel coal into that stove to keep the engine running, sometimes you have to shovel faster when going up the hills and sometimes you have to shovel slower when going down the hills. If you have just the right amount of coal for the job, then there is no extra weight on the train. However, if you have more coal than needed for the job, that excess coal is going to add weight to the train as it loads down the storage car—and someone keeps filling the storage car on a regular basis. If you don't have enough coal in the engine room, then you take some from the storage car and throw that coal into the fire.

Calories are no different. Calories are fuel for your body. The body uses what it needs and stores the rest. If you have more calories than you need, the extra calories (introduced to the body in the form of carbohydrates, fats, or proteins) are converted to fat stores and add weight to your system. If you do not have enough readily available calories, then the body takes those fat stores and converts them to usable energy. It is impossible to perfectly balance your caloric intake with your energy needs on a daily or even weekly, basis. The key is to run a relative balance over the course of weeks and months to maintain your current weight.

When you are trying to lose weight, you need to run a deficit so your body uses some of its stored energy (fat) and reduces your weight. It is that simple. Just like the steam engine, if the storage car is filled with coal, you can start to burn that off and fill it less frequently until it's down to the right size.

Your energy needs are determined by a multitude of factors, including your level of activity (exercising vs. sitting vs. sleeping), your basal metabolic rate (yes, you can blame your weight on a slow metabolism), your body composition (pound for pound muscle will cause you to burn more calories than fat because muscle is a contractile, and thus energy-consuming, tissue), the temperature of your surroundings, and even gender, to name a few. Some of these factors can be altered (exercise to increase your level of activity, build more muscle mass, etc.) while others are less flexible (gender, basal metabolic rate). Basal metabolic rate can be altered, at least to an extent, by increasing your muscle mass.

Your energy intake, however, is much simpler. Barring medical procedures with intravenous (IV) lines and feeding tubes, calories can only be taken in via your mouth. This line of intake is, as you already know, completely flexible and controllable. Maintaining control of this intake, while a challenge, is possible with the appropriate dose of self-discipline, knowledge, and understanding. Thus we will focus on increasing your energy needs (exercise) and decreasing your energy intake (diet). Alas, it all comes down to diet and exercise.

Before we embark on this journey, let's dissect some of the

popular (or unpopular) diets that have been introduced in the past and look at the theory behind these diets and the pros and cons of each diet.

Atkins

The Atkins Diet was (and remains) a popular, broadly followed diet that looked at our intake in terms of the way our bodies react to the food we eat. Until this diet came along, it was generally accepted that your body fat was in direct correlation to your fat intake. There were hundreds of diet programs and books that told you to cut out fat and if followed, you would lose fat.

Atkins changed the paradigm of diets. He put forth, supported with strong evidence, that limited carbohydrate intake would force your body into a state of ketosis, which means your body is using its fat storage as an energy source. Most of us know someone who has had success with this diet, and there is little doubt that it can work for many people. However, it also can create unhealthy fluid shifts within the body especially in the short-term, resulting in muscle cramps, headaches, and fluctuations in weight.

As well, there are drawbacks to this diet that limit its effectiveness as a long-term weight loss solution. The main challenge many have seen is the inability to maintain the strict limitation on carbohydrate intake. Because the system relies more on metabolic actions as opposed to total caloric intake (although you will see later than meat and protein are not exorbitantly calorie dense as compared to other foods), a slight misstep has a much greater negative impact on weight loss or maintenance than a diet that is based on a more balanced caloric intake.

From personal experience, I found that on Atkins I would lose the weight on a strict carbohydrate-limited diet until I reached a goal, and then I would relax a little, then a little more. I was quickly back to the starting point. I never knew quite how much to eat. It was easy to go from cheating a little to cheating a lot because the difference between small carbohydrate amounts and large amounts was minimal.

In other words, a little slipup was nearly as bad as sitting down to eat an entire cheesecake. Couple this with the high fat intake associated with low-carbohydrate diets and there is a high possibility of your weight going up and down, which we can all agree is not healthy. As we lose weight, we often metabolize or break down muscle along with fat, especially if we are not exercising our muscles adequately. When we gain weight, it predominantly comes back as fat stores. Thus, as your weight cycles up and down, no matter which diet program you may be using, you may be slowly substituting your muscle with fat. I may be wrong, but I do not think anyone sees that as a goal.

So how does this fit into the ProportionFit diet program? It offers us a great tool when thinking about the food we eat. It should not be assumed that low fat equates to weight loss or healthy eating. In fact, have you ever noticed that some candies advertise being a "fat-free food," as if that makes them healthy? Simple carbohydrates are sugar, and sugar consumption is the most immediate cause for your body to store energy in the form of fat. On the other hand, a diet consisting of only protein and fat is not reasonable either. A balanced diet with moderate amounts of carbohydrates, protein, and fat that allows you to satiate your wants without derailing your weight loss is the goal of the ProportionFit diet. Bring on the carbs, fat, and protein (all in moderation) and you will experience a sensible and workable weight management program.

The Zone Diet

Popularized by author and biochemist Barry Sears, this program looks at the division of carbohydrates, protein, and fats in a 40:30:30 ratio. Taking some lessons from the Atkins diet, this ratio is designed to allow your body to work at its most efficient level, maximizing the depletion of your fat stores while also creating an environment for muscle development.

While the Zone is certainly based on sound scientific principles (in the ProportionFit Diet we recommend a relative goal ratio of one-third carbohydrates, fats, and proteins, which is quite similar and easier to remember but is certainly not a strict edict), it is not specifically designed for weight loss. The Zone diet is actually more about eating what they consider the "right" ratio of food types and giving your body the correct metabolic zone to work at peak efficiency. When we take some of the good points from the Zone program and blend them with our ProportionFit portion management system, the result will be a healthy and more appropriately sized you.

The South Beach Diet

This diet program is based on three phases of weight loss and food "allowances." The initial phase involves eliminating starches and sugars, similar to the Atkins diet. The second phase is more moderate in its restrictions, and the third phase is more liberal in what one can or cannot eat. Again, this is a good diet overall (developed by a cardiologist, after all), but it defines the food categories based less on calories and more on food types, which may affect your blood sugars and overall health. In general terms, the ProportionFit Diet is similarly designed, with a simple one-third division of carbohydrates, fat, and protein as a recommendation.

Volumetrics

This diet involves eating a full meal, filling your stomach to its desire. However, instead of limiting the volume of what you eat, you are encouraged to eat foods with "low energy" contents or high water content (such as lettuce, celery, and similar foods). This serves to fill you up but delivers fewer calories to your bloodstream.

Again, this is certainly a sound principle because the whole basis is to limit your calorie intake. In the Volumetrics case, the volume of what you eat may be the same as your usual diet, but the calorie content of that food is deliberately lower. In the ProportionFit Diet, the volume of the food you eat is lower than your regular diet, but because the food is "average" with regard to calorie content (it is the same food you normally eat), you will see an overall reduction in your caloric intake.

The Portion Plate

The Portion Plate is a simple means by which the dinner plate is embossed with information regarding proper portions in an effort to give you a visual reminder of what to eat and how much. However, it does not take into account the individual's size or weight loss goals. Once more, this is a sound principle but does not address an individual's goals or current weight.

Many other fad diets exist, including the Paleo diet, *Good Calories, Bad Calories*, the HCG diet, different detoxes and cleanses, along with many, many others. While these are all well intended, the ProportionFit diet is designed to be exceedingly simple and effective for weight loss and healthy weight maintenance without confusing formulas, gimmicks, expensive plans, or supplements.

If you want to get more protein in your diet, take some lessons from the Atkins, South Beach, and Zone Diet programs. If you want to increase your fiber intake, understand the Volumetrics principles. If you want to visualize your division of portions (starch, fat, protein, etc.), go with the Portion Plate. However, if you want to keep it simple, read on and follow the ProportionFit Diet and couple it with a healthy, fresh diet from Subway.

In summary, all of these diet plans have good concepts to consider and embrace. However, they involve either complex changes to your diet or systems that are costly and/or cumbersome. With the ProportionFit plan, you do not have to change what you eat significantly; you just have to manage the volume of intake. That's it. We'll help you with that shortly.

Here is one more way to look at the ProportionFit concept: When you fill your car with gasoline, do you measure the potential energy in the gas or just the volume (gallons or liters) of gas? Unless you are really into physics, you probably just measure the volume. And you also know about how far you can go with each gallon of gas. The distance traveled may vary slightly based on the high octane (think: fats) versus the low octane (think: protein and carbohydrates), but on average you know how far you'll go based on each gallon you add to the tank.

Your proverbial gas tank/digestive system can be thought of the same way. Instead of measuring the potential energy in the food consumed (calories), measure the calories you consume based on the volume of food. Forget counting calories; count cups—just like filling your car's gas tank.

Chapter Three Bottom Line:

Consider again this hypothetical scenario. Imagine going back in time to one year ago and eating exactly the same food items you ate all year long, but cutting out 10% of the volume of food you ate. Same food, just 10% less. Your weight today would be approximately 10% less than it is now. Let's use that same concept moving forward to lose 5%, 10%, 20% or even 50% of our body weight in the next year or months. No matter the magnitude of your goal, it is attainable. This is not a fad. It is based on real science and real results.

Life is pain, highness. Anyone who says differently is selling something.
—William Goldman, *William Goldman: Four Screenplays*

CHAPTER 4

Why "Fad" Diets Do Not Work and Are Not a Solution

If you have ever attempted a diet in the past and failed, you are not alone. Most diet fads come and go because they are not sustainable solutions. They are either not practical (you just can't have bacon for every meal, Atkins' fans) or not based on sound principles (a balance of intake and output). A fad is a temporary fashion or craze followed with extraordinary enthusiasm by a group. The key element to that definition is the word *temporary*. Fad diets are temporary solutions whereas most dieters are not interested in temporary solutions, unless you're just trying to get into a bikini for your vacation in the Caribbean.

The old-fashioned solution of diet and exercise is based on sound principles and permanent weight control. For example, when I read *The South Beach Diet*, I was struck by the testimonials, which had a common theme: statements about how easily individuals lost weight and then regained some weight but were convinced they could easily lose the weight again if necessary. Many of the principles of *The South*

Beach Diet are sound (the author *is* a cardiologist after all), but the formula is less than intuitive and difficult to maintain in today's society.

As well, a diet that gives you a sudden weight loss at the start may seduce you into thinking you will always be able to shed the pounds quickly and safely. Thus, this is the reason for the testimonials about regaining weight but being convinced they could easily lose it again. The problem is, when you think something is easy, you'll always decide to do it tomorrow. And as Annie so eloquently put it, tomorrow is only—and always—a day away. If you work on your weight management now, slow and steady is more likely to win the weight-loss race and provide a sustainable solution.

Fad diet solutions are often touted as painless or they will tell you that you can eat more and weigh less. As the adage goes, if it sounds too good to be true, it probably isn't true. To lose weight, you need to change your routine. Change can be good, but it may cause you to be hungry on occasion, and that's okay. In our age of abundance, it is easy to over consume. There is food all around us. We are genetically programmed to store excess energy as fat because food was not historically this abundant (think: nomads). Today we don't have to go more than ten minutes without a meal or a snack within arm's reach. So go ahead, be hungry on occasion. That is just a signal from your stomach and your body that more calories are wanted. Show that stomach who is boss, and let it find its calories elsewhere and deplete some of those fat stores. This is not a starvation diet, just a controlled intake diet.

Chapter Four Bottom Line:

Science and past performance proves the ProportionFit Diet to be sound and effective. This is not a fad.

Striving for success without hard work is like trying
to harvest where you haven't planted.
−David Bly

<u>*Testimonial*</u>*:*

*"Thank you for giving us The ProportionFit Diet.
Using the philosophy of your book, along with
moderate exercise, has allowed me to lose 10 lbs. in the
first two months of 2014. This wouldn't be such a great
accomplishment except that I have been trying to lose 5
pounds for over a decade!
Thank you for the simplicity and "doability" of your
plan. I have recommended your book to many of my
friends and relatives. Your plan succeeds where other
plans fail, because of its common sense approach and
ease of use."*

*Thanks again,
-Anonymous*

CHAPTER 5

Understanding Calorie Intake

The simple deficit of 3,500 calories can result in the loss of approximately one pound of weight or body fat. Similarly, the additional intake of 3,500 calories can result in the addition of one pound. Thus, the concept is simple: reduce your caloric intake through deliberate limitation of calories to have a *calorie negative* balance (fewer calories are digested than utilized). However, counting calories is far too complex to be practical on a daily basis. The introduction of Deal-a-Meal (for old-school dieters), Weight Watchers, low-carbohydrate diets, and just about any other diet has been intended as a solution to the complexity of calorie counting. Nobody can take the time to count the calories in every meal. It is just not practical. Unless you only eat pre-packaged foods that have defined nutritional information, you cannot realistically count every calorie.

Thus enters the ProportionFit Diet. By averaging the calorie count in common foods and assuming a relatively balanced diet (i.e., don't eat cake and ice cream for every meal), we can generally count the calories in each meal by measuring the size of the meals. While this method may not be accurate to the exact calorie, absolute caloric precision is not necessary. We are dealing with the big picture here. In limiting your calorie intake, and hopefully increasing your calorie expenditure through additional exercise, you will achieve your desired goal of weight loss and improved health.

The reality of our typical food intake is this: whether you eat pizza, a hamburger, pasta, or a steak and baked potato, the volume of what you eat dictates the calories, not just the type of food. If we use a mixture of high calorie–dense foods (meat, pasta, desserts, etc.) with low calorie–dense foods (most vegetables, some fruits, etc.) and control the volume of intake, then we can better balance our diet and calorie intake.

Here is one more way to think about calorie intake to give it perspective. Imagine your metabolic system is like a campfire. As that campfire is going strong, you can put a fairly sizable log on the fire and it will burn, albeit slowly. If you continue to put large logs on the fire, however, there will be a lot of unburned wood in the fire pit.

That is analogous to the extra calories given to your internal camp fire—your metabolic system. However, if you continue to feed that fire with small branches and sticks, given at regular intervals, but only enough to keep the fire burning as hot as you want, that fire will continue to consume (burn) that wood and the large logs placed earlier, leaving nothing but ash.

This should be your food consumption mantra: take in enough to keep the fire burning. If you have extra weight to lose, that weight is like that extra wood you put in the fire pit a while ago. As long as you keep the fire burning, eventually that log will be consumed and reduced to ash. Adding small bits of wood to the fire will help it burn faster. Starving the fire or embers of any wood (or starving yourself of calories) will not allow that fire to burn hot and turn that log to ash. Blowing on the fire is like exercise—giving the system a little oxygen to burn hotter and faster.

Chapter Five Bottom Line:

Calories come in by way of the cup: Count cups, and you will count calories. There is no simpler way.

The way to get started is to quit talking and begin doing.
—Walt Disney

<u>Testimonial</u>:

"I'm in my mid sixties and I finally found an eating program that works for me. I have struggled with being overweight my entire life, and have tried every diet ever published. I would be somewhat successful on each of them, but always put the weight back on. I discovered The ProportionFit program 15 weeks ago and I have lost 30 pounds. I don't think of this as a diet. For me, it's a way of eating for the rest of my life. It is so simple. All you need to do is visualize cups and count them. I still have 70 pounds to lose, but I know I will make it and keep it off with ProportionFit.
Thanks Nick for creating this method."
–Kathy

CHAPTER 6

Understanding Basal Metabolic Rate or Resting Metabolic Rate

Based on a few factors, it is fairly simple to determine your basic calorie expenditure during the course of an average day. In other words, how many calories do you need daily to function? This has been worked out through formulas taking into consideration your weight, height, age, and sex and has been termed the Basal Metabolic Rate (BMR) or Resting Metabolic Rate (RMR). This calculation does not take into account your activity level and is merely the base calorie requirement for your body to function. For consistency, we'll refer to this as the BMR. While the formula may be somewhat complex, many opportunities to calculate this number are available online. Some of these sites include: bmrcalculator.org and bmi-calculator.net/bmr-calculator/.

For example, a 250-pound, 30-year-old male who is six feet tall and has an average activity level has a calculated BMR of approximately 2,200 calories. As you determine the BMR, using weight as the only variable, you can see the graphical representation of an individual's BMR and how it declines simply because he or she weighs less (figure 1). After all, it takes more energy to move a 250-pound frame around through a day's activities than it does to move a 150-pound body.

Also, keep in mind that these averages are for a 30-year-old person and of only basal activity levels. If you are younger or older, your caloric needs can be relatively higher or lower, respectively. Similarly, this does not take into account any activity level; thus, your activity level will increase your energy demands from this baseline.

Figure 1: BMR examples

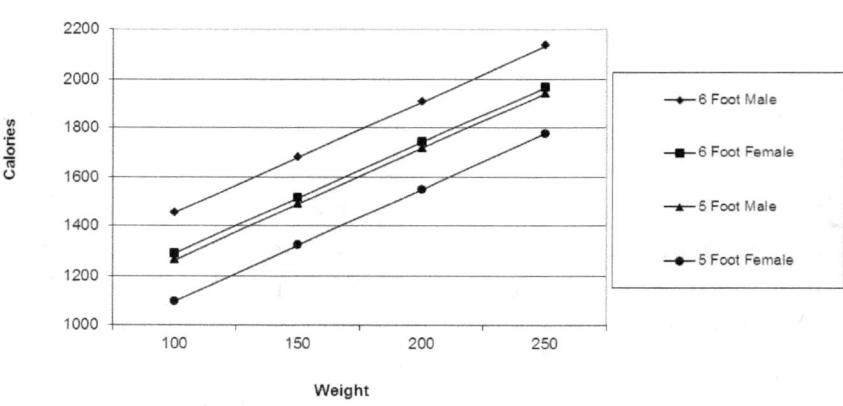

Figure 1: A comparison of basal metabolic rate (BMR) for 30-year-old males and females

In *figure 1*, note the difference in BMR for males versus females and also based on height and weight. As age increases, the energy requirements also will slowly decline. It is also noteworthy that a 6-foot, 250-pound male requires approximately twice as many calories as a 5-foot, 100-pound female (approximately 2,100 vs. 1,100 calories, respectively). In the same context, the difference between a 100-pound female and a 150-pound female is only about 250 calories. That's less than two cans of regular (sugar) soda daily. Thus, weight gain or loss can be simple, tricky, subtle, frustrating, easy, and rewarding all for the same reason—it doesn't take much.

To reiterate, these numbers do not correlate exactly with the calorie requirements mentioned in this book (14 calories per pound). The BMR calculation involves basal calorie requirements and essentially no activity, whereas the ProportionFit calculation is kept simple and assumes a mild to moderate level of activity (reality). The BMR calculation also takes height into consideration, while the ProportionFit calculation ultimately does not bother with height when determining calorie needs.

Finally, note once more the difference between males and females. In general, females require about 100 to 200 calories fewer than males at the same weight. In the ProportionFit Diet, we are not making a distinction between male and female to keep it simple. While this is a real difference in calorie requirements and should be kept in mind, the amount is small enough that we will ignore it when calculating our calorie and cup requirements.

Chapter Six Bottom Line:

Your nutritional requirement is defined primarily by your current weight. Similarly, your body is programmed to take in enough calories to sustain itself based on your current weight. To lose weight, you must consciously and deliberately take in the appropriate number of cups (calories) to lose weight and then, once your goal weight is achieved, maintain your goal weight. Without understanding this simple concept, most individuals overeat, causing weight gain. That weight gain leads to a higher calorie set point, additional overeating, and further weight gain. This concept breaks that cycle.

The truth will set you free, but first it will piss you off.
—Gloria Steinem

CHAPTER 7

Problems Associated with Obesity

While the potential medical, societal, and psychological problems associated with obesity are too numerous to mention comprehensively in this book, a few of the common conditions are mentioned here to track your progress during your weight-management program. Weight management is not just about seeing a lower number on the scale; it is more about feeling better physically and mentally, living longer and healthier, and giving yourself an edge. If you suffer from any of these conditions, look for them to improve as your weight loss progresses.

Sleep apnea: One of the common consequences of obesity is the development of sleep apnea, which is the temporary cessation of breathing (and oxygenation of your blood) during sleeping. This can be due to the increased tissues in the airway causing the occlusion of the airway when sleeping. This results in a disjointed sleep pattern and deoxygenation of your blood, which leaves you tired, lethargic, and thus less likely to be active during the day. This can create a vicious cycle of lethargy, causing decreased activity, leading to increased weight gain and further difficulties with sleep apnea. It can also result in a sharp elbow to the ribs waking you at night as your spouse is startled by your loud snoring or irregular breathing.

Lethargy: While lethargy may be a result of sleep apnea, listed above, it may be a primary result of obesity. The simple work required to move a 300-pound body versus a 150-pound body is greater not just for your peripheral muscles but your heart, lungs, and all systems. Avoiding this work (i.e., not moving), which may be deemed lethargy, is the natural reaction to obesity and the increased workload required. Fortunately this can be reversed with weight reduction. Losing the weight will put that spring back into your step that may be otherwise missing. After all, when is the last time you saw an obese person skipping down the road?

Diabetes: Diabetes, or the body's inability to adequately regulate blood sugar, can be a result of obesity. While not all diabetes is caused by weight gain, obesity can increase the risk of developing this condition, which in turn can lead to increased difficulty in maintaining a healthy weight. Conversely, weight loss often allows the body to improve its ability to regulate blood sugar. In fact, many diabetics will find themselves no longer requiring medication (or at least requiring less) when they lose excess weight and improve their overall health.

Arthritis: Arthritis in the form of wear and tear on your joints (primarily the knees and hips) can often be the result of excess weight loading the joints during activities, whether simple walking and standing or more strenuous actions. Unfortunately, once this wear has developed, it cannot be reversed. However, weight loss can help greatly by either preventing the wear from occurring in the first place or taking the stress off of already-worn joints.

Self-esteem: So much focus is placed on weight through the common media that it is not difficult to see a link between weight and self-esteem or feelings of self-worth. While there is certainly nothing wrong with feeling comfortable or confident with the body you are in (after all, most of us cannot reach the supermodel physique), an even better alternative is to work on our bodies to bring them into the normal range of body mass index (BMI). Not only will this remove the stigma related to being overweight, but it will also empower you with the knowledge that you do have control of your weight and the ability to define yourself as you see fit.

Chapter Seven Bottom Line:

Getting yourself to a healthy weight has multiple benefits. Experience those benefits by following this simple program. Your mind and body will thank you.

Life's hard. It's even harder when you're stupid.
—John Wayne

CHAPTER 8

Physiology 101

Stupid is such a harsh word, Mr. Wayne. However, we could all learn something and benefit from a little education throughout life, including what makes us tick. Our diet and physiology, while natural and instinctual, are areas most people know little about. After learning these tips and secrets, my goal was to share them with everyone else in a condensed and easy-to-understand format. Part of that includes an understanding of the basic physiology related to diet, exercise, and the digestive system to make sense of why this plan will work. It is one thing to hear how diet and exercise can help in weight loss; it is another thing to understand why diet and exercise can help. Commence with the understanding!

When you read food labels and the percentages listed on these nutritional labels, these numbers are usually relative to a 2,000-calorie-per-day diet. This number was developed somewhat arbitrarily by the United States Department of Agriculture (USDA) and adopted by the Food and Drug Administration (FDA) in determining the Recommended Daily Allowances (RDA) of certain components of foods (proteins, fats, carbohydrates, and certain vitamins and minerals). As a rule, however, this 2,000-calorie diet is appropriate for individuals ranging from an active 8-year-old male to a sedentary 25-year-old female to an active 80-year-old female. In other words, it captures a wide range of individuals as an estimate of appropriate daily calorie expenditure and requirements.

Figure 2 shows the USDA "MyPyramid" food and caloric intake guidelines broken down by age, sex, and activity level. In this table, you will see the significant variation in caloric needs based on these simple factors. Thus, we do need to individualize caloric intake based on your age, sex, and activity level to get a better understanding for your true daily caloric expenditure and intake. You may also note that the calorie intake for anyone, male or female, active or sedentary, does not vary by more than 200 percent above age 12. Above this age cutoff, the minimum calorie requirement (75-year-old sedentary female or 12-year-old sedentary female) is 1,600 calories. The highest calorie requirement, in the active 20-something male, is 3,200 calories.

Keep in mind that the simple acts of sitting, breathing, and sleeping all burn calories, and therefore an obligatory caloric intake and expenditure occurs even without significant activity. When you raise that activity level through exercise or other vigorous activities, your caloric expenditure rises significantly, allowing you to develop a calorie-negative balance much easier. In fact, with vigorous exercise, it is possible to raise your daily calorie requirements (expenditures) well above 5,000 calories per day. Then you'll really feel the (calories) burn.

The USDA "MyPyramid" guidelines make the assumption that the individuals are of average and appropriate weight. However, we cannot make that assumption. Based on others' research, the average person needs about 13 to 15 calories per pound of body weight. Higher activity levels will push that requirement up to 15 to 20 calories per pound, whereas lower activity levels may bring the level down to 10 to

13 calories per pound. To keep the estimate clean, we will assume that the average person will require approximately 14 calories per pound of body weight. This makes the calculation simple and reproducible. Always exact? No. Let's not get mired down in the details.

MyPyramid Food Intake Pattern Calorie Levels

MyPyramid assigns Individuals to a calorie level based on their sex, age, and activity level.

The chart below identifies the calorie levels for males and females by age and activity level. Calorie levels are provided for each year of childhood, from 2-18 years, and for adults in 5-year increments.

	MALES				FEMALES		
Activity level	Sedentary*	Mod. active*	Active*	Activity level	Sedentary*	Mod. active*	Active*
AGE				AGE			
2	1000	1000	1000	2	1000	1000	1000
3	1000	1400	1400	3	1000	1200	1400
4	1200	1400	1600	4	1200	1400	1400
5	1200	1400	1600	5	1200	1400	1600
6	1400	1600	1800	6	1200	1400	1600
7	1400	1600	1800	7	1200	1600	1800
8	1400	1600	2000	8	1400	1600	1800
9	1600	1800	2000	9	1400	1600	1800
10	1600	1800	2200	10	1400	1800	2000
11	1800	2000	2200	11	1600	1800	2000
12	1800	2200	2400	12	1600	2000	2200
13	2000	2200	2600	13	1600	2000	2200
14	2000	2400	2800	14	1800	2000	2400
15	2200	2600	3000	15	1800	2000	2400
16	2400	2800	3200	16	1800	2000	2400
17	2400	2800	3200	17	1800	2000	2400
18	2400	2800	3200	18	1800	2000	2400
19-20	2600	2800	3000	19-20	2000	2200	2400
21-25	2400	2800	3000	21-25	2000	2200	2400
26-30	2400	2600	3000	26-30	1800	2000	2400
31-35	2400	2600	3000	31-35	1800	2000	2200
36-40	2400	2600	2800	36-40	1800	2000	2200
41-45	2200	2600	2800	41-45	1800	2000	2200
46-50	2200	2400	2800	46-50	1800	2000	2200
51-55	2200	2400	2800	51-55	1600	1800	2200
56-60	2200	2400	2600	56-60	1600	1800	2200
61-65	2000	2400	2600	61-65	1600	1800	2000
66-70	2000	2200	2600	66-70	1600	1800	2000
71-75	2000	2200	2600	71-75	1600	1800	2000
76 and up	2000	2200	2400	76 and up	1600	1800	2000

*Calorie levels are based on the Estimated Energy Requirements (EER) and activity levels from the Institute of Medicine Dietary Reference Intakes Macronutrients Report, 2002.
SEDENTARY = less than 30 minutes a day of moderate physical activity in addition to daily activities.
MOD. ACTIVE = at least 30 minutes up to 60 minutes a day of moderate physical activity in addition to daily activities.
ACTIVE = 60 or more minutes a day of moderate physical activity in addition to daily activities.

United StatesDepartment of Agriculture
Center for Nutrition Policy and Promotion
April 2005
CNPP-XX

USDA

Figure 2: USDA MyPyramid Table

(From U.S. Department of Agriculture. ChooseMyPlate. gov Website. Washington, DC. Accessed March 2013.)

All of this talk of calories necessitates an understanding of our friend the calorie. Calories, in nutritional terms, are scientifically known as "kilogram calories" or "kilocalories." Without getting into too many details, calories are a measure of energy (we will use "calories" throughout this book to refer to nutritional calories, which are the same as kilogram calories). One calorie is the amount of energy required to raise the temperature of one liter or kilogram of water by one degree Celsius. One gram of fat contains approximately 9 calories, whereas one gram of carbohydrates or proteins contains approximately 4 calories and alcohol, 7 calories. Therefore, gram for gram, fat provides more than twice the energy of protein and carbohydrates.

This can result in easier weight gain if you unwittingly take in too many fatty foods because the same volume of fatty foods will provide more than twice the calories as the same volume of carbohydrates or proteins. Fiber, by definition, is a food component that is not fully absorbed by the digestive system and provides much of the bulk of the stool produced. Thus, fiber is an important part of your diet not just from a nutritional standpoint but as a means of keeping your digestive system working smoothly and efficiently by providing bulk to move the food components through the stomach, small intestine, large intestine, and rectum (not that you need to spend too much time thinking about all of those details).

Component of Food	Calories per gram
Fat	9
Protein	4
Carbohydrate	4
Alcohol	7
Fiber	0*

*Fiber contains the potential energy of other carbohydrates, but this goes unprocessed by your body and results in a zero-calorie designation

Figure 3: Food components and their caloric content

When you eat that Twinkie or piece of pizza, you begin the digestive process by first breaking the food down into smaller pieces through chewing and introducing some of the digestive enzymes through your saliva. The process continues in the stomach and small intestine as the food is further broken down chemically to absorbable components. Once absorbed into the bloodstream, the body then breaks these components (fats, proteins, carbohydrates) into usable energy through one of two primary energy-producing cycles. If that energy is not immediately necessary, these food components are then transformed into the production of fat, muscle or other tissues (brain, liver, kidney, etc.).

Fat stores are the body's efficient way of saving reusable energy for the future, when a meal isn't readily available. This is arguably a wonderful evolutionary adaptation from centuries ago when nomadic humans went for days between meals; in today's society, it is difficult to go hours without seeing a fast-food restaurant! Food used to be for survival; now food has become entertainment, gratification, and a social event. Comfort food did not exist in the good old days when humans were hunting or foraging for every meal. Back then we had to eat to live; now we seem to live to eat.

The rapidity with which your digestive system absorbs and processes those potential calories depends on the food type. Simple sugars (carbohydrates) are absorbed more rapidly than complex carbohydrates. Proteins and fats are processed even slower than carbohydrates, creating less dramatic fluctuations in your blood sugar levels (which can be quite beneficial for those with diabetes).

In general, a diet composed of approximately even calories from fat, carbohydrates, and protein is a healthy option. We'll call this the *1/3 Rule* because one-third of your calories will come from each of those three categories. As we put this *1/3 Rule* into action, this will be used as a general guide, not a strict edict. Certainly a diet of about 50 percent carbohydrates with 25 percent fat and 25 percent protein would be reasonable as well. The ProportionFit Diet is not about finding a special zone. The primary goal is to limit our caloric intake while spreading out the calories among fats, proteins, and carbohydrates. Our primary weight-loss goal will be to take in fewer calories than those expended. This will be referred to as a *calorie-negative* balance and will result in weight loss because your body has to turn to its fat stores for the needed calories and energy. In comparison, maintaining a steady weight will be achieved with a calorie-neutral diet (equal calories taken in as burned). Weight gain results from a *calorie-positive* dietary balance.

Another way to understand calories is to view them as potential energy units, which is easily demonstrated when looking at exercise. When you move your body through a mile, it requires energy, just like driving a car. Depending on how you move through that mile (such as running, walking, or skipping), that method of movement will determine the amount of energy required.

There are two main differences between running, walking, and skipping: the additional amount of work required to move your body up and down while running or skipping (not much up and down movement with walking) and the difference in the time required to cover that distance. Consider the difference between walking 4 miles in an hour or running 8 miles in that same hour. With running, you have effectively doubled the caloric expenditure in that hour because you have moved your body mass twice as much by running in the same hour it took to walk 4 miles. More on exercise in a later chapter.

Chapter Eight Bottom Line:

Calories are calories are calories. Do not focus too much on what you eat. Just eat a balanced diet. You will focus on deliberately measuring the volume of food you eat and, in doing so, you will lose weight or maintain a healthy weight. Guaranteed.

CHAPTER 9

Eating and Addictive Behavior

Being overweight is undeniably multifactorial, resulting from a mixture of environmental (family traditions, foods available, attitudes about food, etc.), psychological (eating to relieve job or home stresses, poor understanding of nutritional balance, etc.), and natural (your sex, medical conditions, age, etc.) elements. The ProportionFit system intends to help you with your understanding of nutrition and your ability to recognize and identify stresses or other factors that contribute to overeating and empower you with the courage to get yourself to a healthier weight and self.

Part of identifying problem areas involves understanding the potentially addictive nature of eating and the manner in which many of us use food to relieve stress. The parallels between chronic overeating and alcoholism or smoking are numerous, including the continuation of overeating despite the fact that you may have identified a problem.

The primary difference between these conditions is this: you need food to survive, whereas alcohol or cigarettes are nonessential. There is no option for going "cold turkey" or avoiding food altogether. The other difference is this: those who overeat have outwardly identifiable characteristics (obesity) that alcoholics or smokers do not have. Thus, prejudice enters the equation. An alcoholic drinking a beer at the bar usually goes unnoticed; an obese person sitting at the Dairy Queen eating a sundae gains disapproving glances and rolling eyes.

The fairness of this situation is debatable, but the reality is undeniable: we literally wear obesity on our skin, and unfortunately, society may react unfavorably to this fact. We can either choose to change all of society or change the shape we're in. Changing all of society is a tall order for an individual; let's work on the shape we're in and get *ProportionFit*. By controlling our food intake and increasing our energy expenditures, the management of our weight and health is in our hands. Unlike the alcoholic, who cannot just cut down but needs to quit completely, together we can get our food intake to a controlled and appropriate level.

Chapter Nine Bottom Line:

Food intake has never before been quantified so simply as in the ProportionFit Diet. Using this simple tool, we can control our intake deliberately and predictably. Without the right knowledge of food volume intake, the task was impossible. Now, with this simple knowledge of food volume intake, the mission is possible.

It is never too late to be what you might have been.
—George Eliot

<u>Testimonial</u>:

"When I first joined, I was physically active and in pretty good shape, but still struggled with lugging around extra weight. The ProportionFit Diet helped me lose 20 pounds; which I have been able to maintain and keep off for 6 months and counting."
-Katie

CHAPTER 10

Understanding Body Mass Index (BMI)

BMI is the estimated calculation of body composition based on height and weight. Based on this calculation, you can be placed in one of five categories: underweight, normal weight, overweight, obese, or extremely obese. While it is not a perfect tool to calculate your absolute health, it provides an excellent guideline for attaining and maintaining a healthy weight. For example, an extremely muscular or a very unfit male could both be six feet tall and weigh 225 pounds. Based on the BMI charts, either individual would be considered obese while in reality only the unfit male would truly qualify as obese by most practical standards. Thus we are dealing with averages, and slight variations in your body composition can be considered. However, if you are Mr. or Ms. Universe, you probably should not be reading this book or be worried about your BMI calculation. On the next pages you will find the table outlining the approximate BMI for any given height and weight (*figure 4*). Your goal, should you accept this mission, is to get yourself into the normal range. If you do not feel comfortable getting to that level, chose a reasonably attainable weight somewhere in the overweight column. This will be our working goal.

Now that we have a better understanding of BMI as well as an understanding of the MyPyramid table (which generically outlines daily calorie needs), with some tweaking, we can combine the two and determine what your goal caloric intake should be to get to your ideal weight. It's time to get ProportionFit!

Chapter Ten Bottom Line:

BMI is an imperfect tool, but provides some general guidance. Use it to give yourself motivation and a visual tool to lose weight and achieve a healthy BMI.

Body Mass Index Table

	Normal						Overweight					Obese										Extreme Obesity															
BMI	19	20	21	22	23	24	25	26	27	28	29	30	31	32	33	34	35	36	37	38	39	40	41	42	43	44	45	46	47	48	49	50	51	52	53	54
Height (inches)												Body Weight (pounds)																								
58	91	96	100	105	110	115	119	124	129	134	138	143	148	153	158	162	167	172	177	181	186	191	196	201	205	210	215	220	224	229	234	239	244	248	253	258
59	94	99	104	109	114	119	124	128	133	138	143	148	153	158	163	168	173	178	183	188	193	198	203	208	212	217	222	227	232	237	242	247	252	257	262	267
60	97	102	107	112	118	123	128	133	138	143	148	153	158	163	168	174	179	184	189	194	199	204	209	215	220	225	230	235	240	245	250	255	261	266	271	276
61	100	106	111	116	122	127	132	137	143	148	153	158	164	169	174	180	185	190	195	201	206	211	217	222	227	232	238	243	248	254	259	264	269	275	280	285
62	104	109	115	120	126	131	136	142	147	153	158	164	169	175	180	186	191	196	202	207	213	218	224	229	235	240	246	251	256	262	267	273	278	284	289	295
63	107	113	118	124	130	135	141	146	152	158	163	169	175	180	186	191	197	203	208	214	220	225	231	237	242	248	254	259	265	270	278	282	287	293	299	304
64	110	116	122	128	134	140	145	151	157	163	169	174	180	186	192	197	204	209	215	221	227	232	238	244	250	256	262	267	273	279	285	291	296	302	308	314
65	114	120	126	132	138	144	150	156	162	168	174	180	186	192	198	204	210	216	222	228	234	240	246	252	258	264	270	276	282	288	294	300	306	312	318	324
66	118	124	130	136	142	148	155	161	167	173	179	186	192	198	204	210	216	223	229	235	241	247	253	260	266	272	278	284	291	297	303	309	315	322	328	334
67	121	127	134	140	146	153	159	166	172	178	185	191	198	204	211	217	223	230	236	242	249	255	261	268	274	280	287	293	299	306	312	319	325	331	338	344
68	125	131	138	144	151	158	164	171	177	184	190	197	203	210	216	223	230	236	243	249	256	262	269	276	282	289	295	302	308	315	322	328	335	341	348	354
69	128	135	142	149	155	162	169	176	182	189	196	203	209	216	223	230	236	243	250	257	263	270	277	284	291	297	304	311	318	324	331	338	345	351	358	365
70	132	139	146	153	160	167	174	181	188	195	202	209	216	222	229	236	243	250	257	264	271	278	285	292	299	306	313	320	327	334	341	348	355	362	369	376
71	136	143	150	157	165	172	179	186	193	200	208	215	222	229	236	243	250	257	265	272	279	286	293	301	308	315	322	329	338	343	351	358	365	372	379	386
72	140	147	154	162	169	177	184	191	199	206	213	221	228	235	242	250	258	265	272	279	287	294	302	309	316	324	331	338	346	353	361	368	375	383	390	397
73	144	151	159	166	174	182	189	197	204	212	219	227	235	242	250	257	265	272	280	288	295	302	310	318	325	333	340	348	355	363	371	378	386	393	401	408
74	148	155	163	171	179	186	194	202	210	218	225	233	241	249	256	264	272	280	287	295	303	311	319	326	334	342	350	358	365	373	381	389	396	404	412	420
75	152	160	168	176	184	192	200	208	216	224	232	240	248	256	264	272	279	287	295	303	311	319	327	335	343	351	359	367	375	383	391	399	407	415	423	431
76	156	164	172	180	189	197	205	213	221	230	238	246	254	263	271	279	287	295	304	312	320	328	336	344	353	361	369	377	385	394	402	410	418	426	435	443

Source: Adapted from Clinical Guidelines on the Identification, Evaluation, and Treatment of Overweight and Obesity in Adults: The Evidence Report.

Figure 4: Body Mass Index Quick Guide (Source: National Heart, Lung, and Blood Institute; National Institutes of Health; U.S. Department of Health and Human Services.)

May you live every day of your life.
—Jonathan Swift

CHAPTER 11

Exercise

Thus far, we have not discussed any of the exercise requirements in detail. This is one of the hardest parts of any dietary plan because it often involves dedicating time and effort to getting out and exercising. In general, moderate or vigorous exercise should be incorporated into your daily life for a minimum of three hours weekly (i.e., one hour a day, three days a week). If you exercise more, you will burn off more calories (in case you hadn't figured that out already). Electronic pedometers to measure the steps you take daily are a great tool to track your activity and calorie expenditure. Giving yourself a goal of taking at least 10,000 steps per day is a wonderful start to boost your metabolism and fitness. However, exercise can come in the form of walking, jogging, biking, lifting weights, aerobics, swimming, yoga, tennis, hopscotch, skipping, spinning class, and just about any other physical activity you enjoy. If you feel like exercise has been hard work, then you have succeeded in burning off calories. Just as it takes effort to control your intake, it also takes effort to burn off calories. The harder you work, the more calories you burn.

Let's break exercise down into three general categories:

Substitution Exercises

This is exercise that is not truly dedicated to physical activity but is substituted or sprinkled throughout your daily activities in lieu of something else. Most people do not have excess time available for exercise. As a solution to this, first focus on changing couch time for exercise time. Instead of adding large blocks of time dedicated to exercise, find times during your day when you are just sitting, waiting, or otherwise sedentary and substitute that time with calorie-burning activity.

This could mean the minute you wait for the elevator is now substituted with a minute climbing the stairs. Or the twenty minutes you normally use to read the newspaper, you now spend reading the newspaper while on a stationary exercise bike. Or how about the thirty-minute commute to work? Use that time for isometric arm exercises to tone your biceps and triceps and sitting isometric crunches to strengthen and tone your abdominal, lower back, and shoulder muscles while driving. (But always do so safely and without distraction; keep your eyes and mind on the road!) Isometric exercise involves firing competing muscle groups or working against a static resistance so that your body part (arm, leg, and trunk) is not moving through any significant range of motion. You are, however, contracting the muscle against resistance and thus toning the muscle, burning calories, and burning fat while building muscle.

Along with these substitution exercises, you need to exercise at least three times per week for at least an hour each time. This is the minimum requirement to achieve your goal weight. In an ideal world, you should exercise vigorously five days per week, each time for one to two hours. These exercises should consist of equal parts cardiovascular exercise and strength training or toning.

Cardiovascular Exercise

Cardiovascular exercise consists of activities that primarily put your heart and lungs to work without fatiguing your extremity muscles (biking, running, elliptical trainers, walking, swimming, etc.). In other words, your heart and lungs reach their maximum capacity before your arms or legs fatigue and give out. These exercises help to increase your lung capacity, lower your resting heart rate, burn calories, and also work to tone muscle.

I would recommend performing the cardiovascular exercise as the first part of your workout to improve the blood supply to your extremities and to enhance your flexibility. Also, do not forget to stretch your muscles before embarking on any exercises to help avoid injury. If you do not feel comfortable starting an exercise regimen on your own, do not hesitate to consult a personal trainer or a qualified individual for assistance.

Wonderful apps and systems have been developed over the past several years to assist people in their efforts to get fit. Pedometers, fitness-tracking apps, and other devices are readily available to help with your weight-loss efforts. Online tracking tools, motivational support, and additional information are available at *ProportionFit.com*. Check it out. Wireless scales that can interface with your home wireless network are also available, making the job of tracking your weight even easier. Finally, friends, family, and other support groups may be instrumental to your success. Studies have shown that, if you share your goals and intentions with those around you, you are more likely to succeed. This is likely due to their positive support when you succeed and their negative support if you cheat or fail. Win or lose, you'll have witnesses, and nobody likes witnesses when they lose. However, everybody loves witnesses when they win!

Strength Training and Toning

Strength training and toning consist of activities that primarily work your extremity and trunk muscles without fatiguing your heart and lungs (push-ups, pull-ups, squats, sit-ups, bicep curls, bench press, etc.). In other words, your arm and leg (or abdominal, trunk, etc.) muscles reach their maximum capacity before your heart and lungs. These exercises help to increase your muscle mass, burn calories, and increase your basal metabolic rate. The more muscle you develop, the more calories you'll burn in your sleep!

Exercise is a critical element to any weight-loss and health-improving regimen for two primary reasons: 1) the calories burned while exercising create a relative calorie deficit, allowing you to burn more fat and reduce your weight, and 2) the muscle mass you develop through exercise will increase your basal metabolic rate and allow you to burn more calories, even at rest. The indirect benefits of exercise, of course, cannot be ignored. These include improved self-image, positive reinforcement toward your goal, better sleeping habits, and more energy during the day. More benefits exist, but you'll find that out shortly as you embark on your weight-loss journey.

Stretching and toning through yoga, Pilates, and other methods are also important and beneficial. Yoga involves much more than just stretching and working your muscles, such as meditation and creating spiritual unity, but we're going to focus on the exercise aspect for now. When holding a pose, you are performing an isometric exercise that involves firing the muscle (often nearly to fatigue) while not moving the limb or body. In some cases this is less stressful on your joints and body, but you have to know your limitations.

One simple example of a typical exercise regimen could consist of a half hour of cardiovascular exercise (elliptical training, jogging, swimming, biking, vigorous walking, etc.) coupled with a half hour of strength training (weight lifting, sit-ups, push-ups, etc.) on Monday,

Wednesday, and Friday. This would be a good maintenance program and would certainly assist with a gradual weight loss. To accelerate the weight loss, one might add an additional day or two per week or increase the time spent on each exercise component by an additional half hour. Keep in mind, your exercise regimen has to start somewhere. It may start out with walking to the mailbox and back and slowly increasing the distance you walk as your stamina improves. Walking in the house, following exercises on a DVD program, joining a health club, signing up for a 5K race, or riding an exercise bike are all acceptable options. The bottom line is this: move your body.

Keep in mind that calorie expenditure, just like calorie intake, can be correlated with weight. Twice the work is done when a 200-pound body is moved versus a 100-pound body. Therefore, twice as many calories are expended to move a 200-pound frame over a mile as compared to a 100-pound frame. The figure on the following page (figure 5) shows the correlation of weight and calories burned for many activities, as adapted from the data compiled evaluating calorie expenditures based on the weight of the individual.

This same data can be broken down by distance. For example, a 100-pound individual running at an average pace will burn about 70 calories in a mile. A 200-pound individual will burn about 140 calories covering that same mile. That amounts to about 7 calories per 10 pounds per mile when running. Walking that same mile will burn about 4 calories per 10 pounds. While the distance is the same, running requires more work as the body literally moves up and down more than when walking, requiring more calories. In essence, it is less *efficient* to run the mile as compared to walking (it requires more fuel in the form of calories to run the mile).

Similarly, using a machine such as a bike to further improve one's efficiency also diminishes the calorie expenditure down to about 2 to 3 calories per 10 pounds per mile. However, when it comes to exercise, our goal should be to burn as many calories as possible. While we may want our cars to be fuel efficient, we want our bodies to burn as much fuel as possible when exercising.

One more point regarding exercise: You will note on the following table that an hour of exercise may burn 300 to 600 calories, depending on your size. As you will find out shortly, that is equivalent to about one to two cups of food. Given the effort involved in not eating two cups of food versus the effort involved in running for an hour, the easy bet is on not eating two cups of food. Better yet, double your calorie crunch by eating two cups less than usual and exercising for an hour. Now you are into the ProportionFit zone!

In the age-old battle of diet versus exercise, understand that diet trumps exercise 100% of the time. If you control your dietary intake, that cannot be sabotaged by a lack of exercise. However, if you exercise diligently, that can be sabotaged by an inappropriate dietary intake. While exercise is important and helpful for overall health and fitness, it is not a great method for weight loss. After exercising, you physically and mentally want more calories to replace the ones spent. However, rewarding your mind and body with food and calories becomes self-defeating if interested in weight loss. You must commit yourself to a certain dietary intake independent of the amount of exercise performed. No exceptions. Your reward for exercise should not be food, but rather the good health and weight loss you desire.

Chapter Eleven Bottom Line:

An appropriate dietary intake can NEVER be sabotaged by a lackluster exercise program when trying to lose weight. Remember that exercise determines your fitness, while diet determines your weight. An intense exercise program is great for fitness but absolutely has to be combined with a deliberate calorie (cup) reduction plan to achieve weight loss.

Activity (1 hour)	160 pounds	200 pounds	240 pounds	Per 10 pounds
Bicycling <10 mph	290	365	440	18
Golf, carrying clubs	315	390	470	20
Walking 3.5 mph	315	390	470	20
Lap swimming	420	530	630	26
Hiking	440	545	655	27
Skiing, Cross-country	495	620	740	31
Racquetball	510	635	760	32
High Impact aerobics	530	665	800	33
Inline skating	550	685	820	34
Singles tennis	580	730	870	36
Running 5 mph	605	755	905	38
Stair climber	660	820	980	41
Jumping rope	860	1070	1285	54
Running 8 mph	860	1075	1285	54

Figure 5: Activities and calorie expenditure per hour based on body weight (numbers rounded for simplicity)

(Adapted from: Ainsworth BE, et al. 2011 compendium of physical activities: A second update of codes and MET values. *Medicine & Science in Sports & Exercise.* 2011;43;1575.)

I've got nothing to do today but smile.
—Paul Simon

CHAPTER 12
Tips and Pitfalls

In my own and others' experience, we have realized a few things that truly can make or break healthy eating habits. While most have already crossed the paths of these troublemakers, sometimes you have to see it in print to identify the problems.

"There is no such thing as a free lunch."

This is inherently true, I've realized over the years. Whether it is simply because I am cheap (yes, I am) or it dates back to our ancestors never knowing when their next meal may be (a more likely reason, in my opinion), I have found that I can seldom pass up a free meal. After all, it is free (i.e., doughnuts brought into the office, your office manager providing lunch for a solid month's work, the holiday potluck, etc.).

While you may not be paying any money for the meal or snacks, you will pay for it in excess calories. The best thing to do is to walk away. Avoid the free lunch or snacks and stick to your diet plan, or at least meticulously limit your portions based on your weight or goal weight. Same thing goes for the all-you-can-eat buffet. Don't try to get your money's worth. It's not a contest to force the restaurateur into regretting letting you in the door; it's an opportunity for you to exercise self-control and limit your intake to keep it within the appropriate volume.

"There is a lot of air in popcorn."

This is a true statement. However, rationalizing that you can have more popcorn, salad, bread, or Cheerios because of "all that air" is self-defeating. Stick to the system (described later), and eat only the volume of food appropriate for your weight or goal weight—no exceptions. After all, on occasion you may eat something that is small in volume but gives you more calories than it should (like chocolate cake). These calorie-dense foods will average out with the calorie-sparse foods. It's all about the averages.

"I am so hungry at the end of a hard day's work."

This is inherently true and expected, as you have been burning calories all day and limiting your calorie intake. Good job! However, now is the time for resolve and commitment. With the ProportionFit program, hunger is expected. This is not a bad thing. Hunger is the body's natural response to signal the need for more caloric intake as the body is starting to metabolize your fat stores (and if you are not exercising, your muscle mass). If you understand the concept of biofeedback, this is the most blatant and easily understood form of biofeedback. Your body is telling you to eat, so you can respond by filling your stomach with excesses of food or just enough to give your body *some of* the fuel it needs. It can use your fat stores for the rest. Stick to the system because you know it is working. Think again of the campfire analogy. Throw a few sticks on the fire and watch them burn. A log will sit, burn slowly, and remain unconsumed for great lengths of time.

One trick that I have found extremely helpful is to take any leftover dinner items and put them in a two-cup container for my lunch the next day (or in the future). In fact, to my wife's dismay, I have a freezer with several two-cup containers of previous dinners. I can take one out of the freezer, allow it to defrost during the day, and microwave it for lunch. No special meals or expense, very little hassle, and I have a healthy, proportion-appropriate lunch readily available. Similar strategies can be applied to breakfast and dinner as well; grow into the habit of knowing the volume of food you should consume versus the amount you want to consume.

"You should not feel hungry."

Wrong! Feeling full or overeating is much worse. With the ProportionFit system, you will find that you may still feel hunger even after you've eaten. This is due to the conditioning of your system and the size of your stomach. The stomach is a muscle with elastic properties, and it can be stretched if it is repeatedly exposed to large volumes of food. Over time, your stomach size and your system will be conditioned to the lesser, and more appropriate, volumes of food. Again, this is *not* a starvation diet. It is a program intended to limit your food intake to the appropriate level for your age-, height-, and sex-appropriate weight. Beware the diets that tell you that you will never feel hunger; hunger is a natural and expected bodily response. Also, be patient. Immediately after eating your meal, you may still feel hungry. Go find something else to do for a period of time, and you'll probably find that your hunger passes in twenty to thirty minutes.

Think of it this way: if someone weighs 300 pounds but is taking in only enough calories to weigh 150 pounds, the body is going to sense a calorie deficit, and this results in the feeling of hunger. When you are not taking in enough calories to meet the requirements of the body you are in, this will result in hunger. That's okay.

"I've been so good, I deserve a break."

While it may be acceptable to give yourself an occasional treat or indulgence, this can become a very slippery slope. Instead of rewarding yourself with food, find some other means of reward. Buy yourself a smaller dress (guys too, if you are into that kind of thing), take a walk, go to the mall, go golfing, etc. Giving yourself some kind of food reward is likely to negate the advances you have made and become quite demoralizing. Sort of like buyer's remorse (regretting having made a purchase, such as a car), this behavior often triggers eater's remorse. Do not let this happen to you. You can sometimes return major purchases; do not plan on returning your food after eating, because that is just not healthy.

"I do so well during the week, but I fail on the weekend."

Any routine that you establish, such as limiting your intake according to the ProportionFit diet plan, is easier to implement when you have a regular schedule. If you work Monday through Friday, you likely have a routine of getting up, going to work, heading home at the end of the day, having dinner, doing random things in the evening, and then going to bed, only to wake the next day and do the same thing. Limiting your intake during this routine becomes simple because it becomes part of the routine. However, on the weekend your days are likely filled with much less structure and much more temptation in the form of sporting events, gatherings, entertainment, and an outright lack of routine. The best way to combat this is to be aware of the challenge, stay strong and stick to the system. The system will not fail you; however, you could fail the system. More on the system later.

"I can't watch my cups when eating out. I get huge servings."

When eating out, ask for a to-go container immediately. This will allow you to divide the portion that you should eat from the portion that you should not eat. Save the extra for the next day or two.

Chapter Twelve Bottom Line:

These are challenges that we all face, no matter what diet you follow. Acknowledging them and preparing for them is the best way to overcome those challenges. Know this: You are not alone.

There isn't a person anywhere who isn't capable of doing more than he thinks he can.
— Henry Ford

<u>**Testimonial**</u>:

"The 10 pounds I lost in the first 6 weeks of the
program have remained off and I am looking
forward to a steady loss from here on out. The
plan is easy to follow when I realized that I could
really eat anything I wanted but within my allotted
cups for the day. I do try to balance my meals as
far as the food groups go but sometimes you just
have to have a hamburger and fries. Easy to
measure it out and fit it in my cup containers.
When I'm done, I'm done. Measuring gives me a
visual cue to know when to stop!
I'm very thankful for the program. The desire to
lose weight with loads of complicated tallying and
removing entire food groups gets overwhelming
and restrictive. You simplified the process and I
can finally see weight loss success in my future."
–Jeanette

CHAPTER 13

Average Calorie Counts for Food

Now that we have discussed all of the finer points of weight loss, physiology, calories, exercise, and the obstacles to achieving that healthy weight, let's get to the proverbial meat and potatoes of the topic: the meat and potatoes. As has been discussed previously, the entire concept of the ProportionFit diet revolves around average foods consumed on a regular basis but managed with the appropriate (proportionate) number of portions.

Unfortunately, nutritional information listed on product packaging can be reported by serving size (an arbitrary quantity), ounces, number of pieces, grams, or just about any other measure related to size, weight, or quantity. If you have ever tried to figure out what this information means and you have been a bit confused, you're not alone.

To the best of our abilities, we have taken many common food items and determined their approximate calorie counts based on a standard *volume*. The volume we have chosen is simply one cup (approximately 237 ml or 8 liquid ounces) because that is used most commonly for liquids and some solids (chips, snacks, etc.). This allows us to extrapolate the appropriate volume of food that should be consumed on a daily basis for a given weight. For example, if you are the average 150-pound person, requiring 2,100 calories daily, this would suggest that you should consume approximately 7.5 cups of food daily (see the detailed explanation on the following pages). This assumes you are not drinking any caloric beverages; otherwise, the caloric beverages are counted against your food volume on a one-to-one (or cup-to-cup) basis.

While many of the values reported here for calorie counts are exact, reality dictates that the true calorie count of one cup of pizza varies widely based on the crust type, cheese type, sauce, etc. However, we are not as interested in exact calorie counts. We are interested in trends and general calorie counts. These measures give us a guideline to work from and a convenient way to compare an equal volume of lettuce versus steak versus chocolate cake.

Finally, don't be wise guy or gal. Packing a one- or two-cup container with pasta and sauce until it's the density of a brick is no longer a valid cup. Eating a cup of potato chips crushed into a fine powder is not the same as a cup filled with uncrushed potato chips. Fill the cup or container with the food item; do not pack the cup. You will only be cheating yourself. As well, some items are just plain difficult to measure (pizza, sandwiches, etc.), so you will need to eyeball these items. Eventually you will develop a knack for estimating volumes of food to the point that you no longer need to measure them. This definitely is not rocket science. Food science? Maybe.

Figures 6-1 through 6-8: Calorie counts by volume (one cup) of assorted food items (additional items can be researched conveniently at multiple websites, including fatsecret.com and acaloriecounter.com):

Figure 6-1: Meat, poultry, and seafood

Food type: Meat, poultry and seafood (primarily fat & protein)	Calories found in 1 cup volume
Beef pot roast	410
Bratwurst	450
Breaded chicken	360
Breaded fish sticks	300
Broiled cod	175
Chicken Cordon Bleu	310
Crab	120
Fried and breaded fish	290
Fried chicken	400
Grilled/roasted chicken	320
Ground beef	340
Ham	365
Lamb	390
Lobster	145
Meatballs	290
Pepperoni	470
Pork	360
Roast beef	360
Sausage	440
Scallops	280
Sea bass	200
Shrimp	200
Steak	340
Tofu	190
Turkey breast	280
Veal	310
Average for meat, poultry, and seafood:	**310**

Figure 6-2: Vegetables

Food type: Vegetables (primarily carbohydrates)	Calories found in 1 cup volume
Asparagus	30
Black olives	150
Broccoli	50
Brussels sprouts	40
Cabbage	20
Carrots	55
Cauliflower	30
Celery	15
Corn	175
Cucumber	20
French fries	480
Green beans	40
Green olives	210
Green peppers	30
Lettuce salad without dressing	10
Lettuce with 1 tablespoon regular ranch dressing	80
Lettuce with 2 tablespoons regular ranch dressing	150
Mushrooms	20
Onion	70
Peas	120
Potatoes	240
Radishes	20
Spinach	10
Tomatoes	30
Zucchini	20
Average for vegetables:	**90**

Figure 6-3: Fruits

Food type: Fruits (carbohydrates):	Calories found in 1 cup volume
Apple	65
Apricots (dried)	310
Apricots (fresh)	80
Banana	250
Blackberries	65
Blueberry	85
Cantaloupe	70
Cranberries (canned)	420
Cranberries (dried)	340
Cranberries (fresh)	50
Dried mango	320
Fig	450
Fresh mango	120
Grapefruit	75
Grapes	110
Honeydew melon	70
Mixed fruit (in heavy syrup)	400
Mixed fruit (in light or no syrup)	100
Mixed fruit (in light syrup)	140
Oranges	85
Peach	60
Pear	95
Pineapple	80
Pomegranate	150
Prunes	380
Raisins	430
Raspberries	65
Strawberries	70
Watermelon	45
Average for fruits:	**170**

Figure 6-4: Grains and pasta

Food Type: Grains and Pasta (primarily carbohydrates):	Calories found in 1 cup volume
Beef ravioli	305
Biscuits (2 medium)	420
Blueberry muffin (1.5 medium)	460
Brown rice	215
Cheese ravioli	285
Cheese risotto	350
Croissants (2 medium)	460
Elbow macaroni (no sauce)	420
Hash browns	300
Lo Mein	310
Noodles	220
Oatmeal	160
Plain muffin (1.5 medium)	480
Ramen noodles (average, varies by preparation)	270
Spaghetti (no sauce)	220
Spaghetti (with ¼ cup sauce)	255
Spaghetti (with ½ cup sauce)	290
Tater tots	300
Wheat pasta	300
White bread (2 slices approximately 1 cup)	130
White rice	205
Whole wheat bread (2 slices approximately 1 cup)	130
Average for grains and pasta:	**295**

Figure 6-5: Mixed food items

Food type: Mixed items/Other	Calories found in 1 cup volume
American cheese	400
Beef enchilada	400
Breaded chicken sandwich (varies by preparation)	450
Cheddar cheese	455
Chicken noodle soup	80
Clam chowder	165
French toast (1.5 regular slices)	240
Fried rice	330
Grilled cheese sandwich (1 sandwich = 1 cup)	310
Grilled chicken sandwich	300
Ham and cheese omelet	370
Ham and cheese quiche	470
Ham and cheese sandwich (1 sandwich = 1.5 cup)	230
Hamburger (with bun) 1 burger = 1.5 cups	200
Hardboiled eggs (1 cup chopped)	210
Hotdog with bun (1 hotdog = 1 cup)	250
Lasagna with meat	390
Macaroni and cheese	380
Mozzarella cheese	400
Noodles with cream sauce (Fettuccine Alfredo)	415
Pancakes (1.5 6-inch pancakes)	265
Pizza, cheese (1 slice approximately 1 cup)	270
Pizza, sausage (1 slice approximately 1 cup)	280
Reuben sandwich (1 sandwich = 1.5 cup)	300
Roast beef sandwich (1 sandwich = 1.5 cup)	240
Scrambled eggs	360
Submarine sandwich, cold cut (3 inch sandwich)	275
Swiss cheese	500
Taco salad	190
Average for mixed items/other:	**315**

Figure 6-6: Desserts and snacks

Food type: Desserts and Snacks	Calories found in 1 cup volume
Cheesecake	560
Cheesecake, chocolate	700
Chex Mix	240
Chocolate cake (with frosting)	460
Chocolate chip cookies	550
Cupcake (approximately 1)	320
Ice cream, chocolate	290
Ice cream, cookie dough	320
Ice cream, Vanilla	290
Oreos® (approximately 8 cookies)	420
Popcorn (no butter)	35
Popcorn (with butter)	65
Potato chips (crushed)	305
Potato chips (not crushed)	160
Snickers Bar® (approximately 10 fun size bars)	800
Average for desserts and snacks:	**370**

Figure 6-7: Beverages

Beverages:	Calories found in 1 cup volume
2% Milk	120
Apple juice	120
Beer (light)	100
Beer (regular)	150
Chocolate Milk	180
Cranberry juice	140
Diet soda, cola	0
Iced tea, sweetened (varies)	90
Iced tea, unsweetened	5
Long island iced tea (contains alcohol)	240
Orange juice	115
Red wine	200
Regular soda, cola	90
Skim Milk	95
Water	0
White wine	195
Average for beverages:	**115**

Figure 6-8: Average calorie counts

Average for all items listed (minus beverages):	260
Estimate per cup given "1/3 Rule":	280

The final estimate is based on the 1/3 Rule of 1/3 fat, 1/3 protein, and 1/3 carbohydrates and is estimated by taking the average calories found in the mixed food items (315 calories/cup), the calories found in fat and protein foods (310 calories/cup), and the carbohydrate food types (averaging 185 calories/cup). Granted, this is an estimate. We may not achieve exact caloric precision with the average cup of food that every individual eats. However, this will give us a good working calorie count on which we can base our portions.

When we put all of this information together, we can correlate body weight to volume of food consumed. In other words, whatever you weigh at this moment, you are consuming, on average, the corresponding volume of food represented in *figure 7*. Remember: 14 calories per pound of body weight. This also suggests that approximately one cup of food is required for every 20 pounds of body weight. Mathematically, it's simple:

20 pounds X 14 calories/pound = 280 calories
One cup of food supplies approximately 280 calories.

Therefore, approximately one cup of food is necessary for every 20 pounds of body weight. It is simple, so let's keep it simple. (The actual calculation was 270 calories/cup; we rounded up to 280 calories/cup to keep it simple.) Thus, the difference between someone with a 150 pound body versus a 170 pound body is simply one 8-ounce serving daily of whatever is consumed. That's it. If you spread that out over the course of four different meals, then it is a matter of two ounces per meal. That is a negligible amount by most standards and yet it can add twenty pounds to one's frame. So: if you ever wondered how you got to the weight you are at, there is the answer. But, there is hope. For as easy as it is for the weight to slowly add up, we can use that same simple formula to shed the pounds.

Chapter Thirteen Bottom Line:

Measuring irregular items is a challenge, but practice makes perfect. Most people find that they can measure food volumes fairly accurately after just two weeks. More information is available at proportionfit.com, as well as *Figure 9* in Chapter 17 .

Weight (pounds)	Daily Calorie Requirement	Daily Food Volume (cups)
100	1400	5.0
110	1540	5.5
120	1680	6.0
130	1820	6.5
140	1960	7.0
150	2100	7.5
160	2240	8.0
170	2380	8.5
180	2520	9.0
190	2660	9.5
200	2800	10.0
210	2940	10.5
220	3080	11.0
230	3220	11.5
240	3360	12.0
250	3500	12.5
260	3640	13.0
270	3780	13.5
280	3920	14.0
290	4060	14.5
300	4200	15.0

Figure 7: Average daily calorie requirement and food volumes for a given body weight

PART II:

The ProportionFit Plan

Everyone has a plan 'til they get punched in the mouth.
—Mike Tyson, American boxer and actor

CHAPTER 14

The ProportionFit System

The ProportionFit System, simply put, involves eating the appropriate volume of food for the weight you want to be. That's it. Others have described eating food volumes equal to your fist, counting calories, restricting your diet to 500 calories, feasting on bacon, taking pills, counting points assigned to foods, etc. We are making it simple and reproducible. After all, an ideal treatment for anything has to fulfill three criteria: be effective, inexpensive, and easily reproducible by anyone. The ProportionFit program satisfies all three criteria. In this case, a portion is a cup. The portion will be the same for everyone, no matter how big or small the individual. The number of portions (cups) will be proportionate to the size you want to be. (More on this later.) It's so simple, effective, inexpensive and reproducible. If I can do it, you can too—guaranteed.

The ProportionFit System does not involve supplements, crash dieting, eliminating carbohydrates or starches, or anything complicated. You will eat the foods you normally eat, trying to balance them so that one-third (1/3) is carbohydrate (mainly fruits, vegetables, pasta, bread, etc.), one-third is protein (some enriched pastas, meat, fish/seafood, some dairy), and one-third is fat (meat, cheese, butter, etc.). But it is not critical to keep that ratio exact or constant. Sometimes you'll go heavy on the pasta and at other times heavy on the meat. It is all about the averages. In fact, half of intake from carbohydrates is acceptable.

To put the system to work, we will take what we have learned from the previous chapters and apply it to our daily routine. For the most part, we are not going to dwell on the exercise aspect of our fitness program. Many options exist, and as described in the exercise chapter, the key is simply to move your body and sweat. Burn those calories every chance you get.

Indulge me for a moment while we discuss a little philosophy. As mentioned in the opening of this book, this diet plan is not just about eating or a diet. It is about freedom—freedom to choose your size and direct your health. But freedom is not all you need. To truly institute change in your life, you need three ingredients:

- Freedom
- Knowledge/awareness
- The will and ability to act

Without all three, you are unable to create a change in your diet, your lifestyle, or your destiny. Imagine being put in a jail cell, being told you are free to do as you please, but the jailer slams the door behind him as he leaves. The jailer granted you freedom, but without the knowledge or awareness that he left the door unlocked, you will remain imprisoned in the cell. On the other hand, if you are cuffed to a chair in the jail cell (your freedom is taken away) but know the door is unlocked and have the will to get out, you will still be imprisoned. As occurred previously without knowledge, you similarly remain a prisoner without freedom. Finally, if you are granted freedom to do as you please and are aware that the door is unlocked, you will remain imprisoned if you are afraid to act and lack the will to escape. However, given the freedom to act, the awareness that the door is unlocked, and the will to walk out the door, you will no longer be a prisoner. You will walk right out of the door, free at last.

Your diet journey is no different. You are given the freedom to eat what you want. With this book, you have been given a simple awareness and knowledge that is reproducible, effective, and inexpensive to manage your weight. Now it is incumbent upon you to provide the will—the will to act and follow the ProportionFit plan to a better and healthier you.

Chapter Fourteen Bottom Line:

You cannot be free to do something of which you are not aware. Not understanding that the volume of food consumed can be measured and quantified, and therefore controlled, has lead to our collective weight problem. This system provides a simple pathway to follow and succeed.

*The advancement and diffusion of knowledge
is the only guardian of true liberty.*
—James Madison

CHAPTER 15

Why the ProportionFit Diet Plan Works

This plan is successful for multiple reasons but primarily because it puts the control back into your hands. You are not relying on some food-management program to pull you through or a magic pill to melt the pounds off. As well, you do not have to make drastic changes, order meals from a special company, or even alter what you eat. You simply need to ensure that what you eat is relatively balanced (the *1/3 Rule*) and that the portions are limited according to your goal weight. (We'll describe that more in the "Getting Started" and "Executing the Plan" chapters.) This will create a calorie-negative system that will bring your weight into the goal range; once you reach your goal weight, your intake will become calorie neutral.

As you get away from the habit of overeating, you'll find that it takes a lot less food volume to give you a feeling of satiety (no longer feeling hungry). This is in part due to your stomach's "stretch compliance" actually reducing. If you imagine blowing up a balloon for the first time, it usually is very difficult. If, however, you inflate and then deflate the balloon and inflate it again, it is much easier. The elasticity of the rubber allows it to stretch, expanding and accepting the air easier the second, third, or fourth time.

Similarly, the stomach is a large, muscle-lined balloon with many of the same characteristics. Muscle fibers have a capacity to stretch passively and contract actively. When they are constantly being stretched, the compliance of the stomach increases. Conversely, if the stomach is not stretched repeatedly, the contraction or tone of the smooth muscle fibers lining the wall of the stomach increases, thereby decreasing the compliance of the stomach cavity. Part of the body's satiety system involves signals produced in response to the stomach expanding and becoming full.

A large part of the gastric bypass surgery that is rising in popularity today involves creating a smaller stomach cavity, thereby physically reducing the volume the stomach can accept when one eats. Part of my impetus to write this book and develop this system was my conversations with people who have undergone gastric bypass surgery. They were frustrated by the fact that, although they were successful at losing weight after the surgery, they could have done the same thing by just eating how they now eat *after* the surgery. After surgery, they are forced to eat small portions and less food because the altered digestive system is no longer able to accept larger volumes. The same end result could be achieved by simply eating those smaller portions initially, without the surgery.

Thus, if you want to choose between spending less than $20 on a book and portion management tool or a $20,000+ life-risking operation, I think you've made the right choice. You *can* make this happen and succeed in your weight-loss goal. You have been given the freedom to eat what you want. This book will provide the understanding and awareness of what to eat. Now, and most importantly, you are providing the will to act and control your weight by putting that knowledge to good use.

Chapter Fifteen Bottom Line:

The volume of food intake is of utmost importance. Don't allow yourself "free foods" that are low-calorie, as they interfere with the ProportionFit Diet's mechanism of resetting your stomach capacity. If your stomach is conditioned to accept a large volume of food, it will expect that large volume. And it doesn't differentiate between spinach and cheesecake. It just wants volume.

Do not put off until tomorrow what can be put off till day-after-tomorrow just as well.
—Mark Twain

CHAPTER 16

Getting Started

No more putting things off until tomorrow. Time to get started. Now. You've already taken the first step toward getting yourself to a healthier weight by purchasing and reading this book. The only other elements you need to provide are:

1. A portion management tool such as a measuring cup

2. A scale to measure your weight

3. The desire to control what that scale tells you

Now you are armed for success.

The portion management tool (PMT) can be just about any food container that gives you a reliable and easy-to-use reference for food quantities. An 8-ounce measuring cup is an ideal measuring device, but it can be a coffee cup, a 12-ounce soda can as a visual reference, or an actual food container. While most of what is reported here is based on a cup (8 ounces), a two-cup container is a convenient portion management tool. Multiple food-container companies (Ziploc, Glad, Rubbermaid, Tupperware, etc.) manufacture quality containers, or you may already have some lying around the house. After a little training, you will no longer need the PMT to determine your food volumes because you will develop a trained eye to know what a cup of food, or two cups, looks like.

The scale becomes critical to understanding the fluctuations that occur in your weight on a day-to-day and week-to-week basis. Do not obsess about your weight. However, work to understand your weight and appreciate the fluctuations that can occur. There are a few keys to using your scale properly so you can rely on what it tells you:

- Always weigh yourself without any clothing or with very light clothing. If you wear a certain amount of clothing, try to keep it consistent so variations in your weight are really you and not your clothing.
- If your scale is not always consistent, weigh yourself three times in a row and take the average number.
- Do not rest your hands on the wall or have any part of your body touching the wall, cabinet, etc., as this will incorrectly reduce the reading on your scale.
- Empty your bowels and bladder prior to weighing yourself.

Now that you have the scale and know how to use it, I want you to weigh yourself at various times during the day, first thing after you awake in the morning, before and after you use the restroom, before and after meals, etc.

This is not something to do for more than a week, but it gives you an appreciation for the fluctuations in your weight that naturally occur. After all, the scale is simply telling you how much your body weighs. The scale does not differentiate between fat, muscle, urine, hydration status, bowel contents, or the hamburger you just ate. All of these things add weight to your system, so do not get frustrated if your weight does not follow a smooth, linear progression toward your goal. You will have ups and downs, but the trend needs to continue in the right direction.

Dehydration will also cause you to lose weight, but this is not the weight you want to lose. When you are dehydrated, your body does not have the appropriate amount of water on board. Be sure to remain well hydrated, and do not allow fluctuations in your water content fool you.

After a few days of getting to know your body and your scale, now weigh yourself every day or every other day, first thing in the morning. This will be your recorded weight. You can track your weight online at *ProportionFit.com* or on the paper table provided at the end of this book. We want as many people as possible to benefit from this diet, so feel free to share a blank page or two with your friends and family. Additional weight tracking system charts can be obtained online at ProportionFit.com.

On this same chart you need to record your height and weight, as well as your BMI off of the BMI chart from *figure 4*. Now choose your goal BMI and weight based on the BMI chart. For many individuals, this may be at the upper end of the normal category, although choosing a weight in the overweight category is certainly acceptable. We do not need to build (or demolish) Rome in one day. Our goal is slow and steady weight loss.

For example, if you are a 6-foot male (72 inches) and weigh 250 pounds, your current BMI is 34. If you chose a goal BMI of 25, your goal weight will be 184 pounds (see "Examples" in chapter 20). This is a lofty, but achievable, goal. The final and critical component involves determining the number of cups of food allowed on a daily basis. We will get to that shortly.

Now that you have determined your goal weight, you need to determine the dietary and exercise components of your plan. Before long, you will be a lean, happy, healthy, and ProportionFit machine!

Chapter Sixteen Bottom Line:

The ProportionFit Diet requires only a few ingredients: You, the knowledge provided in this book, a means of measuring your cups, a scale, and the will to put these together for a positive change.

A friend is someone who gives you total freedom to be yourself.
—Jim Morrison

CHAPTER 17

So, What's in the Cup?

The answer: Whatever you want.

The concept is simple: We know portion control equals calorie control, so let's control our calories by controlling our portions.

Any calorie-containing substance needs to be measured so we can control the volume of food taken in on a daily basis.

In other words, your breakfast cereal, with milk, should be measured and recorded. Your sandwich and chips for lunch—measured. Salad, lasagna, and ice cream for dinner? Measure that too. If you decide you absolutely have to drink a sugar-containing soda, alcoholic beverage, or even a glass of milk, it should be monitored closely and counted against your cup count.

Try not to *drink* more than 200 calories daily. Keep in mind that one of the easiest (and sneakiest) ways to take in too many calories is through calorie-laden beverages. These can consist of regular sodas, alcoholic beverages, juices, sweetened iced teas, and milk, as well as other liquids. Not everything that is touted as being healthy truly is healthy for your system. While milk is a great source of calcium and protein, it also has a few calories that go along with it. Thus, try to stick with water, diet beverages, coffee, skim milk, and tea, while avoiding other sugar-containing beverages. A calcium supplement with Vitamin D may be helpful for most individuals, especially if you limit your milk intake.

Your diet should allow for a wide variety of food types. You don't have to eat celery sticks and water for every meal. In fact, the beauty of this system is the ability to accommodate for whatever you already eat. You do not have to order special meals to reach your goal. Just make or buy whatever you would normally eat (within reason) and keep track of your cups (portions).

Through our research shown previously, we have determined the average calorie amounts contained in a wide variety of foods (including but not limited to spaghetti, lasagna, hamburgers, French fries, bread, steak, fruit, vegetables, chicken, etc.) and utilized the cup as our universal portion size, assuming you will eat a variety of foods. (See *figures 6-1 through 6-8*.)

Thus, while the calories found in a cup-size portion of steak is different than a cup-size portion of chocolate cake or bread, we hope you are not going to submit yourself to an all-cake or all-steak diet. When you buy meals from other diet programs, you are simply buying a controlled-portion meal. (Did you ever notice that these meals never look as big or good as they do on the box?) Eliminate the middleman and the cost while also eating meals you like. Just make sure you follow your recommended number of portions and eat only the quantity of food allowed.

Finally, calorie counts or expenditures will not be the same for everyone (go figure ...). One individual may eat one-cup portions on a regular basis, while another may prefer two cups or three cups of food for a meal. As well, depending on your gender, basal metabolic rate, exercise patterns, and the average calorie content of the food you are eating, you may require slightly more or less food volume on a daily basis than recommended. If you fi nd that the food volume you chose is not achieving the desired goal, reduce the daily portions by one-cup increments until you are seeing the results you need. Some flexibility must remain because "actual results may vary."

Feel free to fill the PMT with healthy foods. We want to encourage that kind of behavior. This can be your favorite homemade lasagna, vegetables, Subway, a hamburger and fries (on occasion), or steak and potatoes. It doesn't matter. What does matter is that you: 1) do not allow yourself to overindulge by eating more than your number of ProportionFit portions, and 2) do vary the food types included in your meals to balance your diet (fruits, vegetables, meats, grains, etc.). That food volume is your limit, divided into at least 4 meals daily. And use common sense. Don't pack the containers with food so tightly that you are, in essence, packing two cups of food into one cup. Don't pack; merely measure or place the food in the container.

How did we come up with the ProportionFit portion? Based on others' hard work, we already know that most people burn about 13 to 15 calories per pound. So if we simply figure that, on average, an individual will burn about 14 calories per pound, this gives us a daily calorie requirement. That part was easy. Determining the manner by which one measures the intake has been a bit more difficult until we stumbled upon a simple truth: a cup of food supplies enough calories for about 20 pounds of flesh. How did this come about? First of all, the cup was a naturally convenient and easily reproducible volume measurement. Then, when we measured and determined the average number of calories found in a cup, we found that the number of calories found in a cup correlates to about 20 pounds of body weight. Thus, for every 20 pounds a person weighs, he or she has to consume about one cup of food. Very simple and easy.

While this is presented as a purely linear equation, the actual formula is much more complex and multifactorial (see previous chapter on BMR). However, for our purposes, this linear relation will suffice. On the following pages you will find a table showing some relative weights and projected calorie requirements. Remember: the assumption for each of these individuals is a normal amount of body fat, muscle, and activity levels. Most individuals will be seeking a goal weight somewhere in the 100- to 250-pound range based on their height and fitness level.

Also note, as mentioned previously, that the ultimate calorie difference between a 100 pound female and a 200 pound male is 200 percent: 1,400 calories versus 2,800. To keep it simple, we will disregard age, BMR, sex, etc. As we age, our activity level and BMR decrease, and that would have to be factored into our daily requirements. However, for simplicity, we will base requirements solely on body weight. Keep it simple.

The reason for using a portion management tool rather than the oft-referenced portions on the package is simple. A portion is normally defined independent of the individual's weight or goal weight. A "portion size" of steak is often cited as being the size of a deck of cards. A potato portion is the size of a tennis ball. According to tradition or precedent, these portion sizes are the same for a 100-pound female and a 200-pound male. In reality, the 200-pound male gets to eat two portions compared to the 100-pounder to maintain his weight and to account for his basal metabolic rate due to that weight. A traditional portion is not proportionate to the individual. However, portion intake should be proportionate to body weight. Instead of varying portion sizes based on body weight, the portion size will be standardized at one cup. The variation will now be allowed as the number of portions (cups) will be proportionate to actual weight or desired weight. Now portions (as a standardized cup) can be used sensibly.

The following figure (*figure 8*) shows the approximate daily calorie requirements based on weight (a repeat of figure 7 previously). This assumes a mild to moderate level of activity and certainly will vary slightly from individual to individual. However, it gives you an estimate of the calories required based on a person's weight. This chart is critical to understand for the ProportionFit Diet (thus, the repetition). In reality, the calorie calculation is just body weight multiplied by 14 calories, and if you recall, approximately one cup of food is required for every 20 pounds of body mass.

One other tip: if you happen to eat something that has a known calorie count, the system can be used in reverse. In other words, if you eat a package of trail mix (one of my personal favorites) that contains 280 calories, count that as a cup of food. If measured, it may only be about 2/3 of a cup. However, if you actually know the exact calorie count, you can go ahead and use the cup equivalent in the daily food volume allowance calculation. Count cups, not calories.

When your PMT is not readily available, determining the volume of food consumed becomes an exercise in practice, practice, practice. In this situation, playing with your food is highly encouraged to determine the exact, or inexact, cup count of irregular food items. As shown in **Figure 9** on the following pages, using handy reference items such as a measuring cup and a 12-ounce can is helpful. However, developing a keen eye for food volume through practice and experience is the ultimate goal. In my experience, most individuals using this system start to develop a knack for estimating food volumes within about two weeks.

Chapter Seventeen Bottom Line:

We're not changing what you eat; we're just changing the volume of what you eat.

Weight (pounds)	Daily Calorie Requirement	Daily Food Volume (cups)
100	1400	5.0
110	1540	5.5
120	1680	6.0
130	1820	6.5
140	1960	7.0
150	2100	7.5
160	2240	8.0
170	2380	8.5
180	2520	9.0
190	2660	9.5
200	2800	10.0
210	2940	10.5
220	3080	11.0
230	3220	11.5
240	3360	12.0
250	3500	12.5
260	3640	13.0
270	3780	13.5
280	3920	14.0
290	4060	14.5
300	4200	15.0

Figure 8: Approximate calorie requirements and food volumes based on body weight (same as figure 7 shown previously)

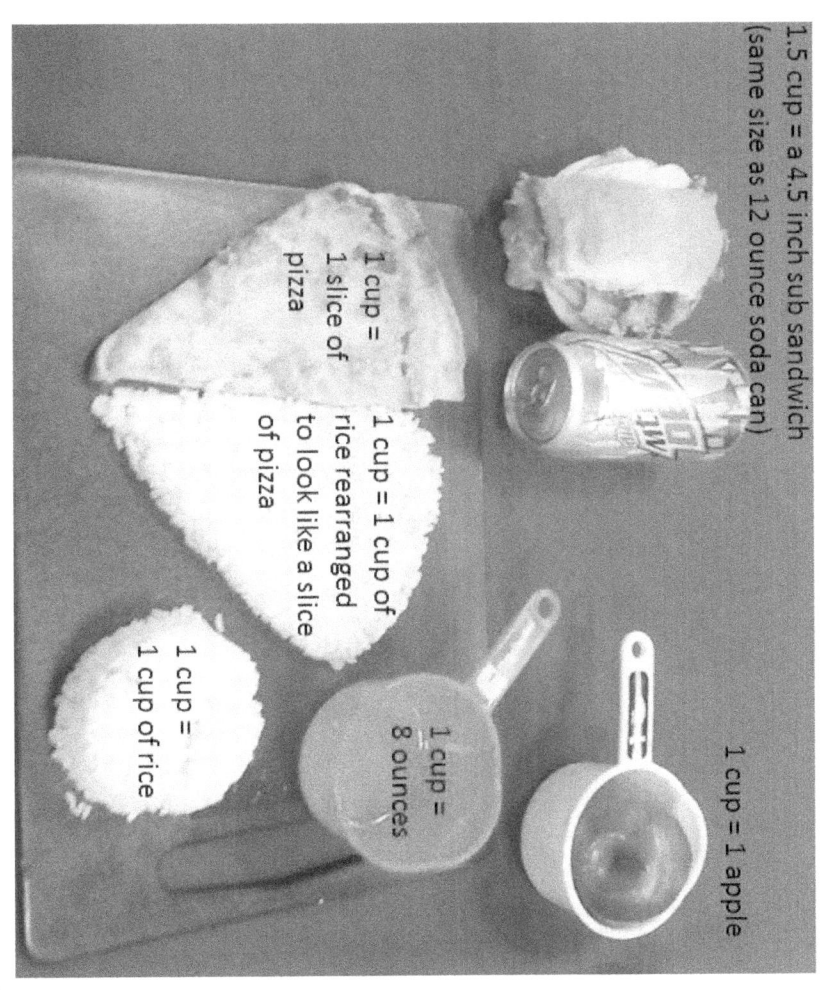

Figure 9: Examples of food measurement with and without a portion measuring tool

1.5 cup = a 4.5 inch sub sandwich (same size as 12 ounce soda can)

1 cup = 1 slice of pizza

1 cup = 1 cup of rice rearranged to look like a slice of pizza

1 cup = 1 cup of rice

1 cup = 8 ounces

1 cup = 1 apple

Dieting is the only game where you win when you lose!
—Karl Lagerfeld

CHAPTER 18

Executing the Plan

Now that you know the concept and ideas behind weight control and exercise, let's put our plan into action. The means by which you use the ProportionFit Diet is up to you and can be placed into one of three categories:

- Maintenance
- Eat to achieve regular weight loss
- Eat to the weight you want to be

Maintenance

Using the ProportionFit Diet to maintain your current weight involves intentionally utilizing your newfound knowledge of calorie content per cup and applying it to your daily consumption. Simply identify your weight on the chart and consume, on average, the number of cups designated that corresponds to your weight. That's it. The volume does not have to be exact on a daily basis but should average the designated volume with the appropriate 1/3 division between fat, carbohydrate, and protein sources.

By consuming, on average, the number of cups of food that correlates with your weight, you will run a calorie-neutral balance and thus maintain your current weight. This may require some fine tuning based on what you eat, but the number of cups consumed should correspond fairly close to your weight. By doing so, your weight should remain relatively constant, and it will help to avoid seasonal and other fluctuations that may otherwise occur.

Eat to Achieve Regular Weight Loss

To achieve regular weight loss, you will consume a fixed number of cups less than whatever is required for your current weight, depending on the rate of weight loss you want to achieve. As we have already learned, for every daily cup deficit, this will lead to approximately ½ a pound of weight loss per week. Thus, after determining the food volume that corresponds to your current weight, you will intentionally consume a number of cups less than that amount to achieve weight loss. However, as your weight reduces (I would recommend adjusting at ten-pound increments), you will similarly reduce the volume consumed according to your weight at that time, always maintaining a 1-, 2-, 3-, or 4-cup deficit (or more). For example, if you weigh 200 pounds, require 10 cups per day, and consume 8 cups per day (a 2-cup deficit), you should lose 1 pound per week. However, always eat a minimum of 4 cups per day as we do not want anyone to consume less than 1000 calories daily. See the following table for additional clarification:

Desired rate of weight loss	Daily intake deficit by cup
½ pound per week	1 cup daily deficit
1 pound per week	2 cups daily deficit
1 ½ pounds per week	3 cups daily deficit
2 pounds per week	4 cups daily deficit
2 ½ pounds per week	5 cups daily deficit
3 pounds per week	6 cups daily deficit

Eat to the Weight You Want to Be

This may be the slowest way to use the ProportionFit Diet program to achieve weight loss, but this approach reduces the amount of calculation necessary. With this approach, you will identify the weight you want to be and eat the corresponding volume of food on a daily basis. While the initial weight loss may be fairly rapid, it will taper significantly as you approach your desired weight. In fact, the last 10 to 20 pounds of weight loss will take years to lose if you strictly follow the diet. Thus, it is often better to use the "Eat to achieve regular weight loss" approach for those final 10 to 20 pounds. With that approach, you could predictably achieve the final weight loss in one to two months.

In general, remember these concepts:

- 14 calories per pound of body weight
- One cup of food = 280 calories
- A 2-cup deficit daily will lead to 1 pound of weight loss weekly
- A 4-cup deficit daily will lead to 2 pounds of weight loss weekly
- Hunger is okay and expected, especially at the outset
- Exercise regularly and progressively, at least three times per week
- Weight loss is reflected by the daily calorie *deficit* at your current weight
- Any calorie containing beverage (including alcohol) should be counted on a cup-for-cup basis against your daily allowance
- Slow and steady wins the weight-loss race

For those interested in losing weight, the program is very simple. The first thing you have to ask yourself is, "How much weight do I want to lose?"

If the answer is less than 40 pounds, then I would suggest using *"Eat to achieve regular weight loss"* approach with a 2- to 4-cup daily deficit to lose weight at a steady pace of 1 to 2 pounds per week, respectively.

If the answer is greater than 80 pounds, then I would suggest the *"Eat to the weight you want to be"* approach, eating the number of cups that correlates with your goal weight. This will involve consuming at least 4 cups fewer than your current consumption (based on figure 8) and will lead to a weight loss of at least 2 pounds per week. With this approach, expect a rapid weight loss initially and a slow tapering of the weight loss as you approach your desired weight. However, once your weight approaches 10 to 20 pounds of your goal weight, then shift to the *"Eat to achieve regular weight loss"* approach for those final pounds.

If the answer is 40 to 80 pounds, then I would suggest using your judgment. (After all, this is about freedom, isn't it?) You could choose to go with the 4-cup deficit for a steady 2-pound weight loss or eat the volume that correlates with the weight you want to be. The former (a 4-cup deficit) will lead to a faster weight loss, but the latter (eat to the weight you want to be) will lead to a slow-and-steady weight loss. Either way, you *can* lose!

To review, here's another table (because you can never have too many tables) for your reference:

Desired weight loss?	Method	Expectations
0-40 pounds	2 cup deficit	Steady 1 pound lost/week
	4 cup deficit	Steady 2 pounds lost/week
40-80 pounds	2-4 cup deficit	Steady 1-2 pounds lost/week
	Eat to the weight you want to be	Initial 1-2 pounds lost per week, slowing as you approach your goal
80+ pounds	Eat to the weight you want to be	Initial 2+ pounds lost/week, slows as you approach your goal

With either of the weight-loss approaches, once you achieve your desired weight, then you fall into the *"Maintenance"* approach to maintain your current weight. It is as easy as (not eating) pie.

Other tips for success:

1. Weigh yourself daily or weekly, at a consistent time of the day, as described in chapter 17.
2. Identify your eating habits, and eliminate your demons (sugary sodas, alcohol, candy, etc.) and limit your nemeses (high-carbohydrate foods such as pastries, pastas, and breads; high-fat foods such as excessive red meats, cheeses, etc.).
3. If you cannot eliminate your nemeses, you may drink 1 to 2 alcoholic beverages or sugar containing sodas/juices daily; however, these must be counted against your daily allowance on a cup-for-cup basis
4. Identify and block out time to exercise, at least one hour for three days a week.
5. Take a multivitamin daily, along with a calcium and Vitamin D supplement.
6. Determine your goal weight based on the BMI chart.
7. Using *figure 8* and your portion management tool, consume only the number of cups allowed daily based on your desired approach (ideally splitting your consumption into at least four meals daily)
8. Include breakfast or a small meal in the morning
9. Never consume fewer than 4 cups per day (approximately 1000 calories)
10. Record your results online at *proportionfit.com* or on the enclosed weight tracking system sheets
11. Watch a new you unfold before your eyes as you dedicate yourself to becoming a healthier, happier, and fit person.

So what if you do not see the results above? The answer is simply this: our calculations are generalities and may not fit your exact scenario. There will be occasions when an individual follows the program and loses weight faster or slower than expected. There will also be occasions when an individual's maintenance volume is higher or lower than the amount reported. By trying to keep the ProportionFit Diet simple, we are not differentiating between males and females, the active and sedentary, or the short or tall. Therefore, adjustments may be necessary. In essence, there can be two common flaws: either your consumption involves food that averages more or less than the 280 calories/cup expected or your daily calorie requirement is higher or lower than predicted (14 calories per pound) or both. If this occurs, simply adjust the volume of intake by a cup at a time or adjust the content (types of foods) appropriately while you continue to use the ProportionFit Diet as a guide. In reality, the greatest criticism for the ProportionFit Diet is also its greatest strength: It is extremely simple. We are not going to account for age, specific activity levels, exact calorie counts, or metabolism. Instead, we will leave that up to the individual to fine-tune their intake accordingly as mentioned above.

Now that you are armed for success, take this knowledge and understanding and put it to good use. You can and will succeed in becoming a healthier individual as you transform yourself into another ProportionFit success story. Better yet, share this knowledge and assist others to propel them on the ProportionFit bandwagon!

See the following examples for our hypothetical ProportionFit participants John Smith, Jane Doe, Pat Johnson, and Chris Smith.

Chapter Eighteen Bottom Line:

Eat the right quantity of food, whether measured or estimated through experience with using a portion management tool, and you will get your weight under control. It is just that simple. And all we needed was a cup and some knowledge all along.

With will one can do anything.
—Samuel Smiles

<u>**Testimonial**</u>:

"Weight loss is easy if you do it your way! I'm down 73 lbs and the weight loss has reduced joint pain by 75%. As I've told you before, I have tried them all, and your book has made the most sense of all the diets out there! I have a goal to run in a 5K race and I think I can do it by next summer.
Thanks again,"
-Anonymous

CHAPTER 19

Examples (John Smith, Jane Doe, Pat Johnson, and Chris Smith)

Profile A: John Smith
Age: 30
Height: 72 inches (6 feet)
Current weight: 250 pounds (BMI 34)
Current food consumption: 12.5 cups/day
Goal weight: 184 pounds (BMI 25)
Goal food consumption: 9.2 cups/day

John Smith is interested in losing weight after being heavier than average for as long as he can remember. Looking in the left-hand column of the BMI table, we find his height (72 inches). Tracking this row to the right to 250 pounds, this column puts his BMI at 34. He would like to get his BMI down to 25. Looking at the top of the chart for the BMI of 25 and tracing this down, the chart shows that this would require his weight to drop to 184 pounds. Then, based on figure 8, John knows that a person weighing 184 pounds will eat approximately 9.2 cups of food in a day.

He wants to lose 2 pounds per week, so he will eat 4 cups less than the number of cups required based on his current weight. Initially that will be 8.5 cups/day because his current weight dictates that he would eat 12.5 cups/day to maintain his current weight. So he makes a goal of eating four meals daily, each one measuring approximately 2.1 cups.

As he loses weight, he will continue to reduce the volume accordingly to maintain a 4-cup deficit, giving him a smooth and continuous weight loss of 2 pounds/week. Once he reaches his goal weight, he will slowly increase his diet back to 9.2 cups/day to maintain his weight at 184 pounds. To track his weight loss, he uses the weight tracking system charts. John writes "250" at the top of the left axis and 180 at the bottom, filling in the intervals between. No one should plan to lose more than 50 pounds in 2 months. In fact, 20 pounds every two months is a lofty but safe goal, depending on your starting weight (figure no more than 2 to 3 pounds per week). In less than a year, John Smith's weight is down to his goal weight!

Also note that, as John begins to approach his goal weight, his weight loss would slow if he did not adjust his intake accordingly. This is due to the less calorie-negative state as one approaches the goal weight and explains why it is always so hard to lose those last few pounds. What works early on (a restricted diet) causes a large calorie deficit early and thus larger weight reduction. Later on as one's weight decreases, the deficit is less drastic, and thus the weight loss is similarly less drastic. Continually adjusting the intake to create a 4-cup deficit (in this case) provides a continuous 2-pound-per-week weight loss. Once John reaches his goal weight, he adjusts his intake to his maintenance level of 9.2 cups per day.

This is an example of *"Eating to achieve regular weight loss"* followed by maintenance once the goal weight is achieved.

Body Mass Index Table

Height (inches)	Normal						Overweight					Obese										Extreme Obesity														
BMI	19	20	21	22	23	24	25	26	27	28	29	30	31	32	33	34	35	36	37	38	39	40	41	42	43	44	45	46	47	48	49	50	51	52	53	54
	Body Weight (pounds)																																			
58	91	96	100	105	110	115	119	124	129	134	138	143	148	153	158	162	167	172	177	181	186	191	196	201	205	210	215	220	224	229	234	239	244	248	253	258
59	94	99	104	109	114	119	124	128	133	138	143	148	153	158	163	168	173	178	183	188	193	198	203	208	212	217	222	227	232	237	242	247	252	257	262	267
60	97	102	107	112	118	123	128	133	138	143	148	153	158	163	168	174	179	184	189	194	199	204	209	215	220	225	230	235	240	245	250	255	261	266	271	276
61	100	106	111	116	122	127	132	137	143	148	153	158	164	169	174	180	185	190	195	201	206	211	217	222	227	232	238	243	248	254	259	264	269	275	280	285
62	104	109	115	120	126	131	136	142	147	153	158	164	169	175	180	186	191	196	202	207	213	218	224	229	235	240	246	251	256	262	267	273	278	284	289	295
63	107	113	118	124	130	135	141	146	152	158	163	169	175	180	186	191	197	203	208	214	220	225	231	237	242	248	254	259	265	270	278	282	287	293	299	304
64	110	116	122	128	134	140	145	151	157	163	169	174	180	186	192	197	204	209	215	221	227	232	238	244	250	256	262	267	273	279	285	291	296	302	308	314
65	114	120	126	132	138	144	150	156	162	168	174	180	186	192	198	204	210	216	222	228	234	240	246	252	258	264	270	276	282	288	294	300	306	312	318	324
66	118	124	130	136	142	148	155	161	167	173	179	186	192	198	204	210	216	223	229	235	241	247	253	260	266	272	278	284	291	297	303	309	315	322	328	334
67	121	127	134	140	146	153	159	166	172	178	185	191	198	204	211	217	223	230	236	242	249	255	261	268	274	280	287	293	299	306	312	319	325	331	338	344
68	125	131	138	144	151	158	164	171	177	184	190	197	203	210	216	223	230	236	243	249	256	262	269	276	282	289	295	302	308	315	322	328	335	341	348	354
69	128	135	142	149	155	162	169	176	182	189	196	203	209	216	223	230	236	243	250	257	263	270	277	284	291	297	304	311	318	324	331	338	345	351	358	365
70	132	139	146	153	160	167	174	181	188	195	202	209	216	222	229	236	243	250	257	264	271	278	285	292	299	306	313	320	327	334	341	348	355	362	369	376
71	136	143	150	157	165	172	179	186	193	200	208	215	222	229	236	243	250	257	265	272	279	286	293	301	308	315	322	329	338	343	351	358	365	372	379	386
72	140	147	154	162	169	177	184	191	199	206	213	221	228	235	242	250	258	265	272	279	287	294	302	309	316	324	331	338	346	353	361	368	375	383	390	397
73	144	151	159	166	174	182	189	197	204	212	219	227	235	242	250	257	265	272	280	288	295	302	310	318	325	333	340	348	355	363	371	378	386	393	401	408
74	148	155	163	171	179	186	194	202	210	218	225	233	241	249	256	264	272	280	287	295	303	311	319	326	334	342	350	358	365	373	381	389	396	404	412	420
75	152	160	168	176	184	192	200	208	216	224	232	240	248	256	264	272	279	287	295	303	311	319	327	335	343	351	359	367	375	383	391	399	407	415	423	431
76	156	164	172	180	189	197	205	213	221	230	238	246	254	263	271	279	287	295	304	312	320	328	336	344	353	361	369	377	385	394	402	410	418	426	435	443

Source: Adapted from Clinical Guidelines on the Identification, Evaluation, and Treatment of Overweight and Obesity in Adults: The Evidence Report.

Name: __John Smith__

Age: __30__

Height (inches): __72__

Starting Weight: __250__

Starting BMI: __34__

Starting food volume (cups): __12.5__

Goal Weight: __184__

Goal BMI: __25__

Goal food volume (cups): __9.2__

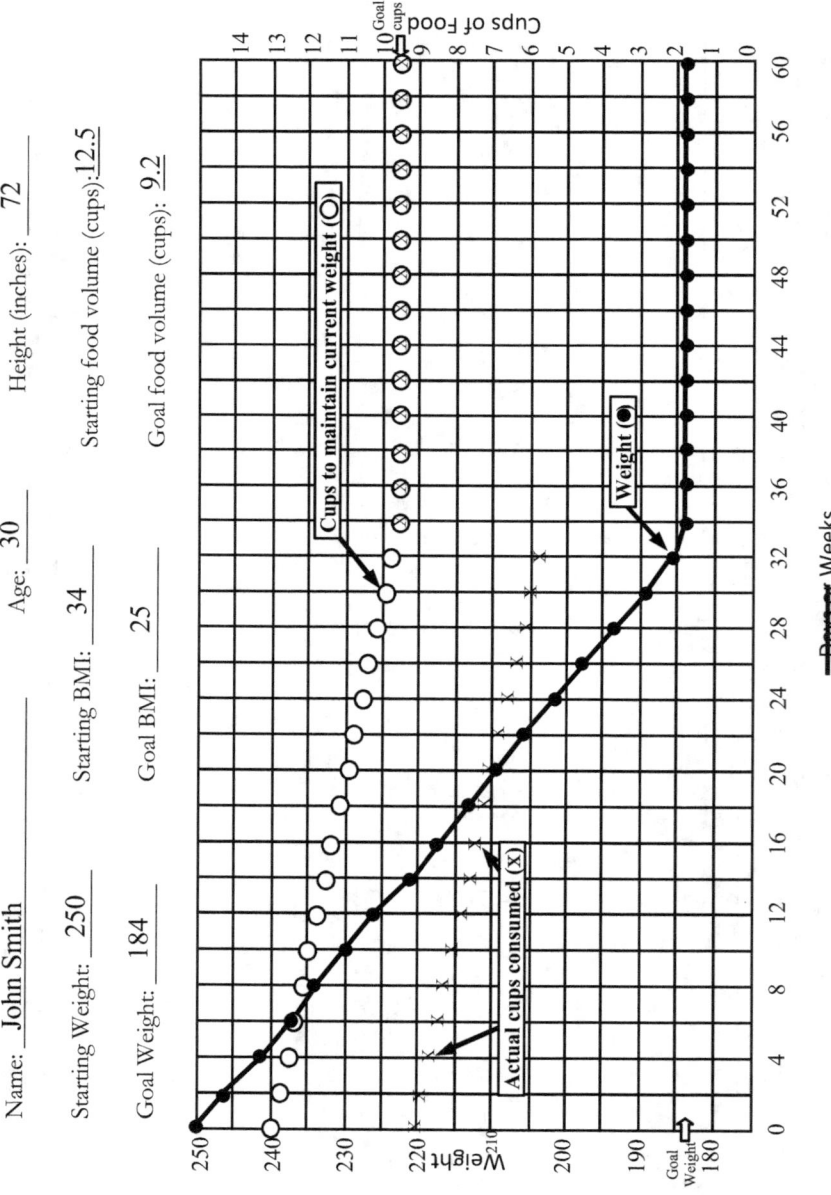

Most folks are about as happy as they make their minds up to be.
−Abraham Lincoln

Profile B: Jane Doe
Age: 45
Height: 66 inches (5 feet, 6 inches)
Current weight: 200 pounds (BMI 32)
Current food consumption: 10 cups/day
Goal weight: 150 pounds (BMI 24)
Goal food consumption: 7.5 cups/day

Once more, Jane goes through the same calculations as John Smith, determining her goal weight as 150 pounds based on her height (getting just into the normal BMI range). Based on that calculation, she knows her daily consumption should be approximately 7.5 cups/day. Her initial calorie deficit will be approximately 700 calories daily (2.5 cup deficit times 280 calories per cup = 700 calories). Thus, she will lose approximately 1 pound every 5 days initially. By increasing exercise (and thus calorie expenditure), she can accelerate the weight loss with the same 7.5 cups/day of food intake.

Rather than maintaining a constant 4-cup deficit like John Smith, Jane's weight loss will be greater initially and slowly taper over many weeks. Thus, unlike John Smith, Jane will still be short of her goal even after one year (52 weeks). As you can see from the weight tracking system sheet for Jane Doe, at 60 weeks the difference between the cups consumed (7.8) and the cups required to maintain the current weight (8.1) is only 0.3 cups. That leads to only an 81-calorie deficit daily, and thus it would take over a month to lose the next pound. In reality, to lose the last 10 pounds, Jane would be better off cutting her intake to a 2-cup deficit (consuming 5.8 cups/day) whereby she will lose about 1 pound per week until she reaches her goal weight.

This is an example of *"Eating to the weight you want to be"* followed by maintenance once the goal weight is achieved.

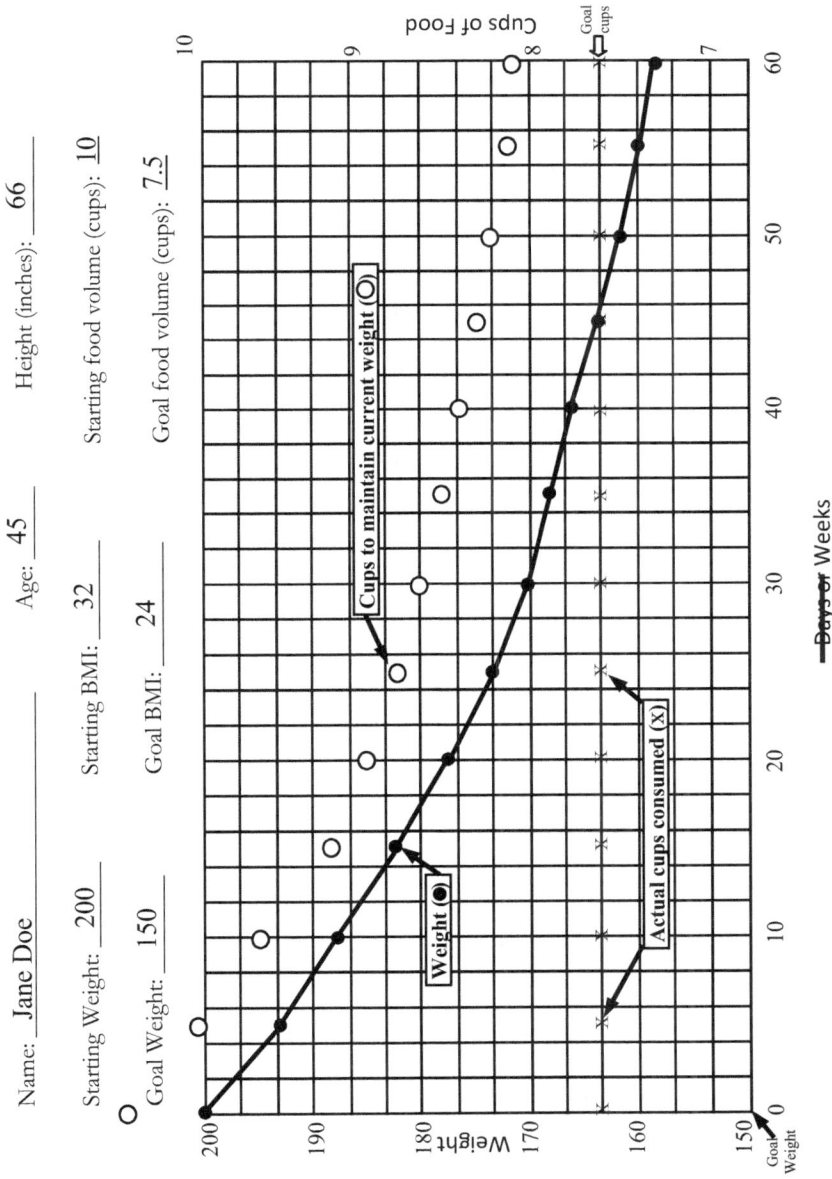

Name: Jane Doe

Age: 45

Height (inches): 66

Starting Weight: 200

Starting BMI: 32

Starting food volume (cups): 10

Goal Weight: 150

Goal BMI: 24

Goal food volume (cups): 7.5

Cups to maintain current weight (O)

Actual cups consumed (X)

Weight (●)

Cups of Food

Weight

Days or Weeks

Profile C: Pat Johnson
Age: 60
Height: 60 inches (5 feet)
Current weight: 300 pounds (BMI >54)
Current food consumption: 15 cups/day
Goal weight: 125 pounds (BMI 24)
Goal food consumption: 6.25 cups/day

For Pat, the goal is to bring the weight down to a healthy range at the top end of normal BMI. This will involve cutting food consumption by over 50 percent (from 15 cups/day to 6.25 cups/ day). Because of the Pat's smaller stature, the overall amount of calorie deficit daily is tremendous initially (8.75 cup deficit daily at 280 calories/cup = 2,450 calories daily), resulting in about 2 pounds of weight loss every 3 days. This may be overly ambitious but would result in a fast initial weight reduction.

As Pat loses weight, the difference will lessen between the number of cups required to maintain the current weight and the number of cups for the 125 pound goal. Once that difference reaches a 4-cup gap, Pat will transition to a steady 4-cup difference until the goal weight is reached, thus combining the approaches of John Smith and Jane Doe. This would certainly be a challenge, as Pat will be consuming only 3 to 4 cups daily in the final 10 weeks of the program. (Remember that the ProportionFit Diet suggests always eating at least 4 cups daily, unlike Pat.) However, the consistent and constant results are a motivating factor as Pat sees the success and ongoing march toward the goal weight.

This is an example of *"Eating to the weight you want to be"* transitioning to *"Eating to achieve regular weight loss"* once Pat has reached the 200-pound threshold, followed by the maintenance program once the goal weight is achieved.

Name: Pat Johnson

Age: 60

Height (inches): 60

Starting Weight: 300

Starting BMI: >54

Starting food volume (cups): 15

Goal Weight: 125

Goal BMI: 24

Goal food volume (cups): 6.25

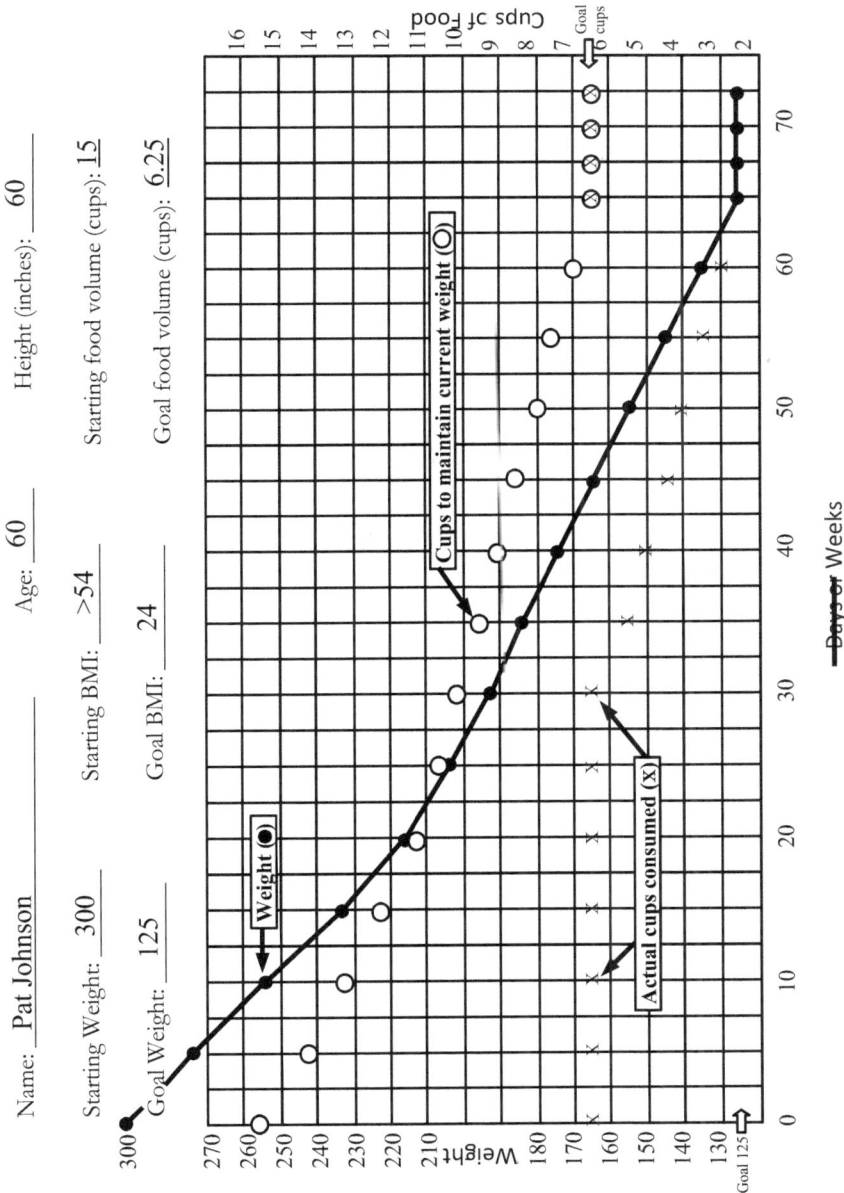

Profile D: Chris Smith
Age: 40
Height: 66 inches (5 feet, 6 inches)
Current weight: 160 pounds (BMI 26)
Current food consumption: 8.0 cups/day
Goal weight: 140 pounds (BMI 23) Goal
food consumption: 7.0 cups/day

It is January 1, and Chris has committed to a New Year's resolution to lose 20 pounds by April. In order to do so, Chris will follow the program with a 3-cup deficit, expecting to lose about 1.5 pounds weekly. Thus, in three months Chris will have lost about 20 pounds by following the program. Initially, the number of cups consumed will be about 5 (3 less than 8 cups), finishing at the end of March by consuming only about 4 cups daily until the goal is reached. This will provide a steady and moderate pace of weight loss, combined with a moderate level of exercise 3 to 4 times weekly to augment the calorie expenditure.

This is an example of *"Eating to achieve regular weight loss"* followed by maintenance once the goal weight is achieved.

Chapter Nineteen Bottom Line:

Many methods exist to lose weight, even within the ProportionFit Diet. Ultimately your goals and personal situation dictate which method is best for you.

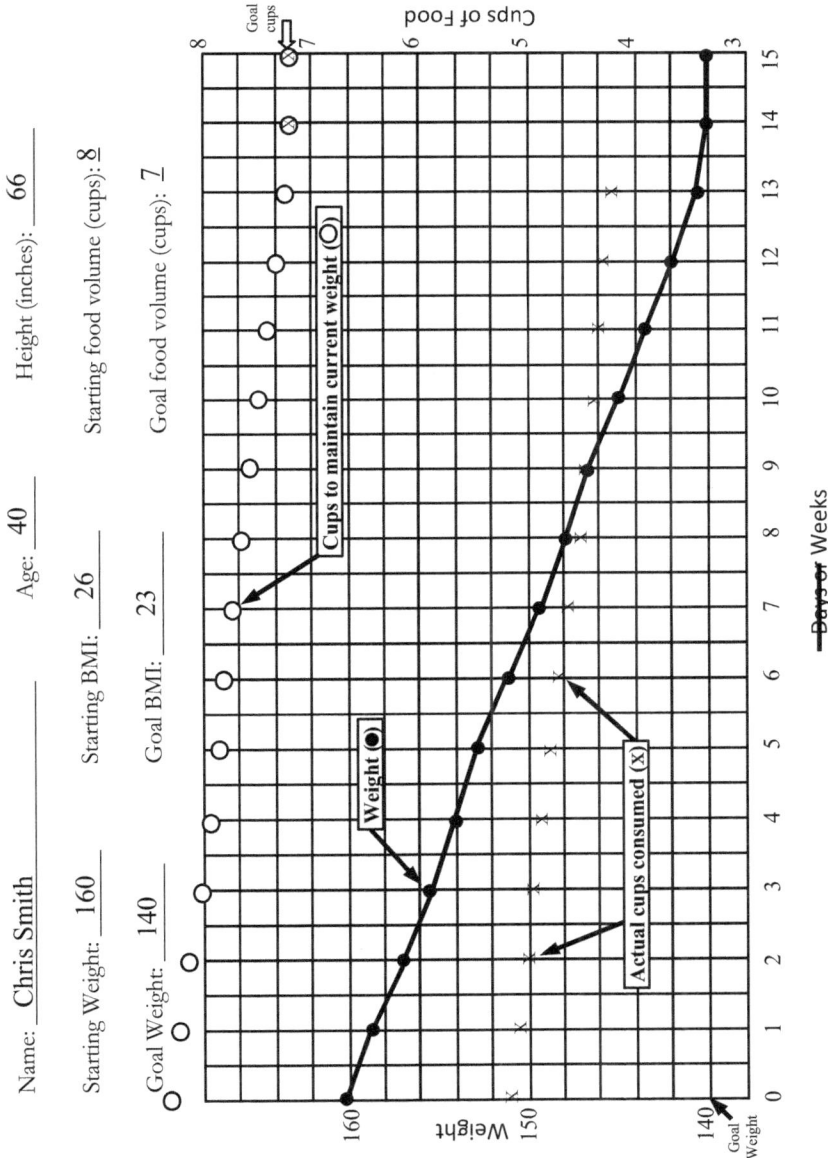

Name: __Chris Smith__

Age: __40__

Height (inches): __66__

Starting Weight: __160__

Starting BMI: __26__

Starting food volume (cups): __8__

Goal Weight: __140__

Goal BMI: __23__

Goal food volume (cups): __7__

<u>**Testimonial**</u>:

"The ProportionFit Diet is the easiest, least expensive, and most productive diet I have ever been on. No extra costs. No calories or points to track. Just follow the diet and you will lose weight. No guilt involved. The results speak volumes."

–Karen

CHAPTER 20

Applying the ProportionFit Diet to Orthopedics

Now that you know everything about The ProportionFit Diet, you may wonder if an orthopedic patient should give their weight and the ProportionFit Diet special attention. The answer is simple: Yes. Patients with a weight above a normal BMI have been shown to be at increased risk of multiple problems, including:

1. Hip, knee and ankle degeneration
2. Spinal degeneration and disk herniation
3. Joint related pain (hip, knee, and ankle)
4. Infection risk after orthopedic surgery
5. Hip joint dislocation after hip replacement
6. Blood clots (deep venous thrombosis [DVT])
7. Gout and pseudo gout (crystalline arthritis)
8. Joint replacement premature loosening
9. Joint mal-positioning during joint replacement surgery
10. Increased cost of joint (hip and knee) replacement surgery

With these risks and potential complications in mind, the importance of a normal BMI (or at least, "overweight" BMI) cannot be overstated. In fact, many insurance companies and government agencies are requiring that patients undergoing a total knee or hip replacement have a BMI at or below a certain level. In many cases, a patient's BMI has to be below 40, 35 or even 30 (depending on the specific requirements in place) for both patient safety and cost. As joint replacement is an elective surgery and, as we have discussed previously, since weight loss or gain is more dependent on diet than exercise, we know that we can help patients lose weight even in light of a severely degenerative joint. The traditional logic and doctor's office conversations went something like this:

> **Patient:** "Doc, my knee hurts so much that I have gained weight. I need a new knee so that I can finally lose this weight I've gained."
>
> **Surgeon:** "You're right. Your knee is worn out and you need a knee replacement."

Unfortunately, as has been shown in many studies, giving an obese patient a new knee or hip does not result in post-operative weight-loss but does put those patients at significantly increased risk of the above-mentioned complications. So, now the conversation goes something like this:

> **Patient:** "Doc, my knee hurts so much that I have gained weight. I need a new knee so that I can finally lose this weight I've gained."
>
> **Surgeon:** "I understand how you feel. However, studies have shown that patients do not lose weight because of their new knee replacement and are at significantly increased risk of infection, poor outcomes, a loose joint, and many other complications, not to mention increased cost. Let's work on getting your weight to a proper level so that we can give you the best outcome possible. While we cannot eliminate all complications related to surgery, we can at least minimize the risks by getting your weight to a more normal level. Once we have your weight to a proper level, then we can proceed with the knee replacement with the confidence that we are giving you the best outcome possible."

This conversation is not unique to knee and hip replacement. Similar results occur with patients undergoing spinal surgery and most orthopedic surgery. While exceptions can and will potentially be made for patients with an elevated BMI, the consensus is to optimize BMI prior to non-emergent joint replacement and spine surgeries.

The best outcome related to weight loss in light of a degenerative knee, hip or back is to avoid surgery altogether. Many patients, after losing weight, will find that the pain related to their degenerative knee, hip or back has decreased significantly, often to the point of no longer requiring a joint replacement or back surgery. After all, the best way to avoid risks of infection, blood clots, dislocation, wound complications, loose joints and other complications related to surgery is to avoid surgery in the first place. Studies have shown that each pound of body weight results in 3-7 pounds of increased stress across the knees and hips, as these joints have small surface areas and thus the force is concentrated across the joint surface. By losing significant weight, patients may experience a decrease of joint pain by 50-90%.

While paying attention to the volume of food consumed is important, the quality of the items consumed cannot be ignored. As mentioned previously, no one is asking that you make drastic changes to what you eat. Your focus should be on the volume of food that you eat. Within those confines, however, we need to pay special attention to nutritional value. For those considering surgery, nutrition is an important factor in the healing process of your surgical wound. Poor nutrition pre- and post-surgery can significantly increase the risk for surgical site infections, delay healing, and impair wound strength. A basic understanding of nutrition and how it can affect the healing process of your surgical site is extremely important.

Protein: Essential for the maintenance and repair of body tissue by promoting collagen development. Not having enough protein can prolong the healing process of the surgical site further increasing the risk of a surgical site infection. Food rich in protein include: meats, fish, eggs, liver, dairy, soybeans, legumes, seeds, nuts, and grains.

Calories: Provides energy and aids in collagen synthesis. If the body doesn't have enough calories to produce energy, the energy will be taken from protein, which may decrease your muscle mass. Proteins then will be used for energy rather than repairing body tissue. Immediately before and after surgery is a critical time to consume enough cups to at least maintain your current weight. This is not the time to try to lose weight by restricting your cup intake significantly.

Carbohydrates: Major source of calories for immediate use by the body and helps prevent other nutrients from being converted into energy. Carbohydrate sources include: whole grain cereals, breads, potatoes, rice, fruits, vegetables and pasta.

Fats: A great fuel for wound healing. It provides the body with fatty acids, a major component of cell membranes. Unsaturated fatty acids must be consumed because the body cannot synthesis enough on its own. Good fats to eat include: Mono- and polyunsaturated fats found in meat, full fat dairy products, and oils and fats used in cooking.

Antioxidants:

Vitamin C: Aids in collagen synthesis and the formation of new blood vessels to help strengthen and heal wounds. It helps the immune system and increases the absorption of iron. Vitamin C deficiency can impair wound healing and can increase the risk of infection. Vitamin C rich foods include: Oranges, grape fruits, tomatoes, leafy vegetables, and fruit juices with added vitamin C.

Vitamin A: Increases inflammatory response in wounds, while stimulating collagen production. If not enough Vitamin A is consumed, deficiency can delay wound healing and increase the risk of an infection. Food with Vitamin A include: Milk, cheese, eggs, dark green vegetables, oranges, and red fruits and vegetables.

Vitamin E: Decrease scar formation and can reduce injury to the wound by controlling excessive free radicals. Foods rich in Vitamin E include: Spinach, almonds, bell peppers, dark leafy greens, sunflower seeds, and asparagus.

Minerals:

Zinc: Important for protein and collagen synthesis, as well as tissue growth and healing. Deficiency in zinc can lead to delayed wound healing, cell growth, and reduced wound strength. Foods with zinc include: red meat, fish, shell fish, milk products, poultry, and eggs. Be careful, too much zinc can actually interfere with the healing of the wound.

Iron: Helps transport oxygen in the blood by way of hemoglobin, aiding in wound healing along with overall oxygenation of blood. Iron deficiency can lead to impairment of wound healing, collagen production, and wound strength, as well as shortness of breath ("iron deficiency anemia" can occur, requiring a transfusion). Iron absorption can increase with the consumption of vitamin C. Foods include: Red meat, eggs, fish, whole wheat bread, dark green leafy vegetables, dried fruits, and nuts. Supplements are also available.

Hydration: Hydration (DRINK WATER!) is a very important factor in the healing of your surgical wound. Dehydration causes the skin to be less elastic, more fragile, and decreases the strength of the wound. It reduces the circulation of blood which impairs the supply of oxygen and nutrients to the operative site. Drink plenty of fluids to prevent dehydration from occurring. Ideally, when urinating, the urine should be relatively clear (not yellow) which confirms that you are well hydrated.

So, the task is simple for patients who are candidates for orthopedic surgery, especially those undergoing total joint replacement: Get your weight to a healthy level. The ProportionFit formula is simple, inexpensive and effective. Simply follow the instructions, watch the weight come off, and get healthy. After losing the weight, if your joints still hurt enough to warrant surgery, then proceed with surgery. However, if the weight loss has diminished the joint pain sufficiently to forego surgery and continue with an active, quality lifestyle: Wonderful. After all, the goal is to improve your health and quality of life through the simplest means possible. It really is that simple.

Chapter Twenty Bottom Line:

Lose weight and your joints will thank you!

119

Always bear in mind that your own resolution to succeed is more important than any other one thing.
—Abraham Lincoln

AFTERWORD

That's it!

We sincerely hope you find *The ProportionFit Diet for Twin Cities Orthopedics* of great use in your weight-loss or -maintenance journey. I, along with many others, have found this to be of significant benefit to maintain and achieve a healthy weight—a health that spills over into everyday life with improved energy, efficiency, strength, and confidence. Please share your successes (or failures—if there are any) with us either in writing or online at ProportionFit.com. You may also track your progress online at the ProportionFit.com website.

Other resources to consider reading for more information:

- *You: A Dietary Guide*
- *Fast Food Nation*
- *SuperSize Me!*
- *Eatright.org*

Go to *www.ProportionFit.com* for more information and resources and to help track your progress. We also welcome any and all comments. Good luck!

Only those who will risk going too far can possibly find out how far they can go.
– T.S. Eliot

WEIGHT TRACKING SYSTEM SHEETS

Name: _____   Age: _____   Height (inches): _____

Starting Weight: _____   Starting BMI: _____   Starting food volume (cups): _____

Goal Weight: _____   Goal BMI: _____   Goal food volume (cups): _____

Cups of Food

Weight

Days or Weeks

123

Name: _____   Age: _____   Height (inches): _____

Starting Weight: _____   Starting BMI: _____   Starting food volume (cups): _____

Goal Weight: _____   Goal BMI: _____   Goal food volume (cups): _____

Cups of Food

Weight

Days or Weeks

124

For additional information and resources, check out:

ProportionFit.com (website),

ProportionFit.info (blog),

and

facebook.com/proportionfit

www.ingramcontent.com/pod-product-compliance
Lightning Source LLC
Chambersburg PA
CBHW060358290526
45791CB00002B/554